Advance Praise for
SLOW FAT TRIATHLETE

"*Slow Fat Triathlete* reminded me why I was captivated by the sport: It has the potential to transform your life. . . . [Williams'] point is that in life, we are all slow, fat triathletes at one time or another, perhaps not literally but as a state of mind. It isn't necessary to lose weight, have your life in order, or have the right equipment to pursue dreams. All that's needed is the courage to start moving in a new direction."

—*Chicago Tribune*

"[A] chatty, inclusive take on [Williams'] journey from obesity to fitness. *Slow Fat Triathlete* is the antithesis of those triathlon training guides on bookstore shelves, the ones written for the tri geeks who already have single-digit percentage body fat. . . . Instead, Williams offers real-world tips on how to cope with chafing or scheduling workouts in a busy schedule."

—*The Oregonian*

"What an enjoyable book! Well written, informative, and inspiring. Go, Jayne, go!"

—Georgena Terry, founder of
Terry Precision Bicycles for Women

"In this provocative, highly humorous, encouraging, as well as realistic and sound guide, Jayne Williams proves that anyone who really wants to can do a triathlon. Way to go, Jayne! You have crossed the finish lines of your races and your book in fine fettle."

—Steven Jonas, MD, author of
Triathloning for Ordinary Mortals
and *The Essential Triathlete*

"Whether you're a tortoise or a hare, a jock looking for new athletic thrills or a jill just trying to get fit, *Slow Fat Triathlete* will get your heart rate revved up by laying out a sensible triathlon training, general fitness, and active lifestyle plan. Ideal multisport reading material for all shapes, sizes, and ages."

—Bill Katovsky, founder of *Tri-Athlete* magazine
and two-time Hawaii Ironman finisher

Jayne Williams

Slow Fat

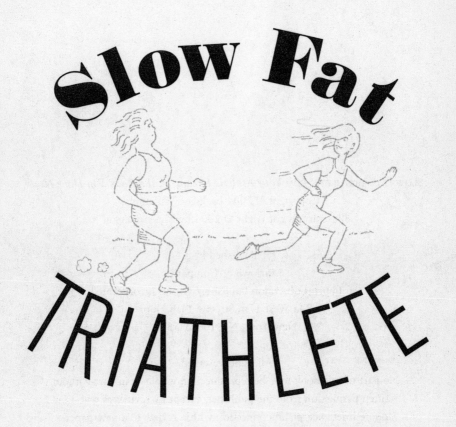

TRIATHLETE

LIVE YOUR ATHLETIC DREAMS

IN THE BODY YOU HAVE NOW

Illustrations by Tim Anderson

Marlowe & Company
New York

SLOW FAT TRIATHLETE: *Live Your Athletic Dreams in the Body You Have Now*
Copyright © 2004 by Jayne Williams
Illustrations copyright © 2004 by Tim Anderson

Published by
Marlowe & Company
An Imprint of Avalon Publishing Group Incorporated
245 West 17th Street • 11th Floor
New York, NY 10011-5300

Library of Congress Cataloging-in-Publication Data is available.

ISBN 1-56924-467-7

9 8 7 6 5 4

Designed by Pauline Neuwirth, Neuwirth & Associates, Inc.

Printed in the United States of America
Distributed by Publishers Group West

To my husband Tim, my parents,

and my brother Jonathan:

You are the core of my world.

This book's for you.

Contents

INTRODUCTION

DON'T BE AFRAID OF THE F-WORD

OH MY GOD, she's using the f-word! Is she calling me fat? Is she admitting to being fat herself? Why would she call herself fat? Or slow, for that matter? What is the meaning of this? Relax. Take a deep, cleansing breath. *Slow Fat Triathlete* is me. I'm a triathlete at a very modest local level. I've been training and racing for two years now. I'm also fairly slow and kind of fat, especially as triathletes go. I used to be a lot slower and a lot fatter, though, and this book is about my journey from injury and obesity to a pretty decent level of fitness using triathlon as my vehicle. It's an invitation to you to come along for the ride, with some tips and encouragement on actually getting started in the sport. My fondest hope is that reading the book will be fun for you, and that you'll close it at the end feeling like you want to go outside and start moving your body around. "Fun" is the f-word that really matters here.

This is not a book about fatties' rights or the politics of obesity or how I'm a victim of the fast-food industry. If you want to read about how overweight folks have a tough time, there are plenty of books out there that can meet your needs. This is not that book. This is also not a book for hard-core Lycra-clad tri-junkies who want yet another training book so they can shave twenty-three seconds off their bike time. If you're one of those people, and you want to read this for fun, that's cool. But don't come back and complain that I didn't make you faster.

This is a book for people like me. Folks who may have struggled with a few extra pounds all their lives, or people who haven't exercised as consistently as they wanted to. Maybe you drive your kids to swim team practice and get a crazy urge to be in that water. Maybe your neighbor did a triathlon and you thought, "Man, you have to be in such great shape to do that." Maybe you're turning thirty or forty or fifty and you have an inkling that you want to accomplish something you haven't done before. This is a book for the Slow, the Proud, the Possibly Fat, Wanna-be Maybe-Someday Triathlete.

If you don't want to categorize yourself as fat, that's just fine with me. But you know, with all the statistics out there about how 80 percent of all Americans over twenty-five are overweight and 30 percent of all of us are obese, I figure that not everyone picking up this book is skinny as a rail. If you don't want to think of yourself as slow, then by all means consider yourself fast. But unless you really are one of those elite athletes who can swim like a seal, ride like Lance Armstrong, and then get off the bike and run like a deer, you are probably going to be in the middle or back of the pack when you start out on the triathlon road.

But here's the thing—you can do it anyway. You can start out fifty or more pounds overweight, with no experience in any of the three sports of triathlon, and you can get yourself to the starting line and even to the finish. You take it slowly and patiently, you accept your limitations even as you push against them, and you commit to being a total and utter beginner, and you can do it.

Being a slow fat triathlete means being a beginner. It's shorthand for anyone who can find it in themselves to do a little training and take part in triathlon at their own pace, on their own terms, for their own reasons, with a mix of pride and humor. You don't even need to be literally fat to be a slow fat triathlete. It's kind of a state of mind. Even if I ever get skinny (unlikely) and fast (really unlikely), I'll still be a slow fat triathlete at heart.

Slow fat triathletes laugh at their foibles, celebrate every step of progress, and measure their success by how much fun they're having, not by medals, and certainly not by prize money. They wear socks with silly graphics, they don't stress about how they look in their race outfit, and they cheer everybody on, whether they're fast or slow. They don't wait until they lose weight or meet some other precondition to get started doing something they want to do.

Slow Fat Triathlete is not a comprehensive guide to triathlons for beginners. I'm not a coach or a trainer or nutritionist or any kind of expert. I want to make you laugh, make you believe you can become a beginner, and point you on the road to your next steps and your next books about triathlon. Hopefully you'll need a whole shelf full.

Oh, and here's a word of advice: Yes, you can hurt yourself doing this stuff. You can get anything from oozing toe blisters to knee problems to a host of nasty injuries if you fall off your bike. If you decide to engage in any of these odd swimming, biking, or running behaviors, do me a favor and check with your doctor, especially if you have some medical condition more serious than a solid set of love handles. And if you fall down and scrape your knee—'cause you might—please don't sue me, OK? Get out the Neosporin and the gauze pads, and watch where you're going next time. Learn the rules of the road and the pool, don't swim alone, run smart, be safe. I'll write a little bit more about this later on.

Jayne

1

LIFE IN THE SLOW FAT LANE

HOW DID I GET HERE?

TRIATHLON 1A

FIRST OFF, WHAT is a triathlon? Most people who hear the word "triathlon" think of Ironman Hawaii, the world championship of triathlon, the most exalted event among triathletes. Ironman Hawaii, held on the volcanic slopes of the Big Island, consists of 2.4 miles of swimming and 112 miles of cycling, topped off by a full marathon, 26.2 miles in usually blistering heat and debilitating winds.

What you may be surprised to learn, though, is that there are different shapes and sizes of triathlon, some of them small and non-threatening, some (though not many) even more intimidating than Hawaii. There are so-called "sprint distance" events, which most of us could not complete at anything resembling a sprint. These tend to be somewhere around a 400-yard swim, a 12-mile bike, and a 3.1-mile run. There are "international distance" races, which are the same distance as the Olympic events. These bump up the ante a little bit to a 1,500-meter swim, a 40-kilometer bike, and a 10-kilometer run. Those international folks and their pesky metric system. That's about a .9-mile swim, a 24.8-mile bike, and a 6.2-mile run, for us Amurrikins. There are half-Ironman races, which just take all the Ironman distances and slice them neatly in half, for those who are only half as crazy as the Ironpeople. And for the extra-insane, there are double-Ironman races. We're not even going to talk about them.

People ask me all the time what the order of the events is. The most usual order is swim-bike-run. I haven't seen this in print anywhere, but it certainly makes sense for safety reasons. Better to be in the water when you're freshest and on your own two feet when you're most likely to collapse from exhaustion.

Despite the undeniable rigors of participating even in a sprint tri, the sport is growing by leaps and bounds. USA Triathlon (USAT), the sport's governing body, reported forty thousand annual members in 2002—more than double the number in 1999. Triathlons are held in city parks and streets, in high mountains and swampy bayous, in France and in Thailand, in New York and Los Angeles. USAT estimates that 150,000 people a year are participating in multisport events now. Most of the folks out there are guys, but a fast-growing number are women. I just attended a small local event where the women outnumbered the men for the second year in a row.

SECRET TRIATHLETE DREAMS

I DON'T THINK everyone should do triathlons. Far from it. Most people just don't see the attraction, and that's fine. I can see where the idea of starting the day with an icy plunge, followed by hours of getting chilled, dizzy, hot, chafed, sweaty, blistered, and exhausted just isn't everyone's idea of a good time. Not that that's really what a race is like, but I think it's what you might think it's like. I don't want people to endanger themselves if they have serious medical issues. I just want to unleash the secret triathlete dreams of people like me, who never thought they even wanted to do this until someone lit the spark in their minds. I didn't know I had secret triathlon dreams, but it turns out I did, and this is my story.

You might think it would be discouraging or depressing to be a 220-pound woman about to start triathlon training, like I was in the fall of 2001. But compared to where I'd been, I was feeling pretty optimistic about it all. Hang with me for a couple pages while I convince you just how unlikely it was that I would ever even start training for a triathlon, let alone work my way up to mediocre results.

There are probably thousands of people out there who have worked their way into triathletehood and overcome far more daunting physical and mental obstacles than I will ever face. My sweaty mesh running cap goes off to each and every one of them. I know how hard it was for me to get to the starting line, with just an average set of problems to manage, and a lot of advantages to help me manage them. I was merely fat, injured, unfit, and approaching middle age.

THE DARK DAYS

WORKING LOTS OF overtime in a cube can really get you fat in a hurry, especially if you like to eat a lot. Always a chunky gal, I was starting to really pack on weight after four years of office life and cheeseburger lunches, and I developed some nasty hand, arm, and shoulder problems from the endless hours at the keyboard. In the summer of 1999, I was thirty-five years old and as far from being a triathlete as it is possible to be. I had had an operation on my shoulder and missed weeks of work with tendonitis in my hands, so I couldn't ride a bike or swim, and, after two years of chronic pain, I'd mostly gotten out of the habit of exercising. And when you spend a lot of time sitting around the house, not able to garden or play guitar or even hold a book for very long, you tend to get bored and depressed. And if you are anything like me, when you get bored and depressed you become a highly evolved cookie-seeking mechanism.

I had chowed my way up to 269 pounds. I was on the verge of not being able to fit in the largest plus-size clothes in the stores, heading for the dubious netherworld of full-figure catalogs, size 4X elastic-waist knit pants and capacious tunic T-shirts. I'm five feet nine inches tall and have always been pretty muscular, so I was one of those chicks who "carry their weight well." This is a euphemism for, "Well, you're pretty fat, but you don't look *that* fat." But you know, I really was that fat. I made myself keep the pictures that prove it.

I don't remember the exact day, but somewhere in June 1999 I decided it just had to stop. I had to learn to eat so that I could get back to a reasonable size, feel energetic, and, most critically, stay that way. I realized that if I didn't change my ways, the magic three hundred number was right around the corner, and who knows where I'd end up? I started the long, rocky campaign to get thinner and fitter while being outside more, and that path has led me to the adventure of being a slow fat triathlete.

WALKING THE WALK

THE FORMULA FOR losing weight isn't very complicated. Expend more calories than you consume on a regular basis. Eat less, exercise more. Four simple words. You'd think I could internalize that. Of course, Einstein's theory of relativity is only $E=MC^2$, and look how hard that is to internalize. So I figured I needed to get some energy going and move my mass. Not quite at the speed of light, but faster than I had been. I started eating energy bars for breakfast and lunch, powering down diet sodas and baby carrots, and eating pretty much a regular dinner. Half the size of my previous regular dinner, I'll admit, but the same basic stuff.

In the shape I was in (roughly that of a small asteroid), the only exercise I could think to do was walking. I still had some leggings that fit me, so my thighs wouldn't ignite from rubbing together, and a couple of XXL T-shirts that hid a multitude of sins. I set out for the suburban sidewalks.

I wasn't totally pathetic. I had done some walking and hiking while I was dealing with my recalcitrant hands and arms, so it wasn't like I was blown out after twenty yards. But I definitely struggled to keep up with my long-limbed boyfriend, and I worked up a good sweat walking a mile. But after a while, I could walk two miles at a pretty good clip, and then three, and even four. I dusted off my YMCA card and started to interact with the weight machines. I did the exercises I remembered from rehabbing my shoulder, and I babied my wrists along as I gripped the handles on the machines.

And you know, the weight started to come off. It really did. I wasn't keeping track, but I know I lost about twenty pounds in the first three months or so. As my upper body got lighter and stronger, my shoulder and hands started to feel better, too. I could ride the exercise bike if I didn't lean too hard on the handlebars, and use the elliptical machines. I kept a close eye on the "calories burned" readouts and tried to burn at least two hundred calories a day. Then I worked on four hundred, then six hundred. I started going to aerobics classes, stumbling through the extraordinarily complex choreography and foreign terminology, working up a determined sweat, trying to face the large woman in the mirror without wincing.

FAT CHICK ON THE RUN

IT STILL DIDN'T seem realistic to think that I would ever be a runner. Even after losing forty or so pounds, I was still pretty hefty, and I thought my knees and feet just wouldn't be able to take the strain. My long struggle with tendonitis also made me think that I was just predisposed to be injured easily and to heal slowly. One of my hand doctors, evidently frustrated with my lack of progress after extensive and expensive treatment, once shook his head and said, "Well, you might just have crappy collagen." Collagen is the healing glue that enables your muscles and ligaments to fix themselves, so this was a depressing thought. A physical therapist with whom I worked described it as "piss-poor protoplasm syndrome." Protoplasm is the goo that carries the collagen. If my collagen and protoplasm weren't good at flowing into little traumas in my tissue and patching it up, would I ever be able to be really active? I had doubts.

I was getting to the point, though, where I had started to notice a little spring in my legs. I'd been strengthening my legs and hips and lower back with weights, and I thought I'd just try jogging a few paces of my usual walk in the park. Careful to stay on soft grass or dirt, I started incorporating a minute of jogging, and then two. My feet creaked a little around the arches, but basically held up. Slowly, carefully, like I was jogging on eggshells, I started padding around the grass a little more. And over time, I managed to run all the way around the park. A little over a mile. I didn't exactly feel like a young gazelle, but I felt I might be able to keep up with an arthritic cow on a good day.

One thing that was inspiring me to get running was that a bunch of my friends were getting into it at around the same time. They all lived an hour away, so we couldn't really get together much and trot around, but just knowing they were doing it too made me feel it was possible. One of the crew suggested we all sign up for a fun run in San Francisco the Sunday after Thanksgiving. Our resident gazelle, Russ, signed up for the 10K race, and we were in awe—6.2 miles! Whoa. The rest of us signed up for the 5K and hoped we wouldn't have to walk too much of the way.

Being pretty much a lazy, procrastinating beach bum at heart, I have always needed a deadline to really get me moving. Now I had one. By

November 28, 1999, I had to be able to run 3.1 miles. I set additional goals of not injuring myself and having fun in the process. I worked my way up to two laps around the park, becoming a familiar, sweaty apparition to the tennis players and dog walkers. And for some reason, three laps weren't much harder than two. I was ready for the run.

The Run to the Far Side is a great way to start a racing career. Gary Larson, the genius behind the Far Side cartoons, is involved with the race and designs the T-shirt, so there's a pretty large contingent of people who dress up like Far Side characters and run the race in the guise of cavemen, or cows, or cats with evil thoughts. There are fifteen thousand people or so lined up at the Porta-Johns before the race, and it's just a nutty scene. Plus, at least half the crowd walks the 5K, so I knew I wouldn't come in last. Russ, Michelle, Chris, Nan, and I reluctantly left our sweats with the sweat-guarding volunteers and huddled for warmth in the foggy morning. My heart was pounding. I had the flight reaction and the fight reaction and the peeing-with-fright reaction going all at the same time. A half dozen fur-clad cavemen shuffled up to the starting line with us, bearing an eight-foot-long carrot and a sign: Early Vegetarians Returning from the Hunt. This was fun. This was San Francisco. This was my first race.

It was a great moment in my life, but it was utterly unremarkable from an athletic standpoint. I didn't finish last. I averaged around eleven minutes and forty seconds per mile, which was way faster than I thought I could go. Turns out you run faster on roads than on grass—who knew? I did beat a couple of the cows, but they were weighed down by their costumes. The cavemen kicked my ass, though, even handicapped by their enormous carrot. It was a fantastic rush to finish the race, and to be going a little faster at the end than I was at the beginning. I felt strong and athletic. I still have the T-shirt, but I gotta admit I still don't actually get Gary's cartoon. Why *did* the Acme moving van run over the tortoise and the hare?

I entered more races, collected more T-shirts, felt a little faster every time. Of course this "feeling faster" is very relative. When I broke eleven-minute miles for the first time, I was ecstatic. To let you know how slow that is, current 10K world record holder Asmae Leghzaoui (isn't that an awesome name? makes me want to be Moroccan) has run 6.2 miles in an astonishing thirty minutes and twenty-nine seconds. That's under five-minute miles. Ms. Leghzaoui would be there and back and I wouldn't even be there yet. Even in a local road race like the Far Side, the winners are running not much over five minutes a mile for a 10K.

I was really dropping weight, too, inching down towards 220 pounds, so I was just around the weight of your average NFL strong safety. At this size, I couldn't run all the time for exercise. I felt like my feet were stressed out. I kept on working the weight machines and the exercise bike, and I even ventured back into the pool. This was a pretty scary step for me, testing my old shoulder and hand problems against the deceptive, slippery resistance of the water. Some pain did resurface, and the whole area of the shoulder joint just seemed weaker and less flexible than it did before a year of pain and a surgery. I guess that would be expected. I swam tentatively, mixing my freestyle with lots of kicking, cautious breaststroke, and even the elegant sidestroke of an old Esther Williams water extravaganza. The shoulder gives me trouble to this day, but I had added another mode of exercise to my arsenal.

A year passed, and I had lost about fifty pounds. I still had no idea of ever doing a triathlon. I didn't know that there were triathlons that people like me could do. My collagen, I firmly believed, was still crappy. But I had made a lot of progress and I was in much better shape. What I really wanted was to ride a bike. I was never an accomplished bike rider, but I used to love taking my mountain bike out for an hour, even sometimes two. But that was before the wrist issues. When I first went to hand therapy, I asked the clinic owner about riding my mountain bike. He looked a little sad and said, "I hope you haven't put a lot of money into that bike." I hadn't, but the implication made me a little sad, too.

I had a germ of an idea infecting my crazed little mind, though. I had seen people cruising around on funny looking recumbent bikes. They're not that common, but in the gadget-crazed geek haven of my Silicon Valley home, intrepid engineers and so on ride them around. I had even seen some that put the handlebars down below the seat, so you could just hang your arms down, relaxing like on your couch, putting no stresses on your hands, wrists, or shoulders. They were extremely uncool looking, but they were wheels. I decided to get one and started doing a little research.

But alas! Disaster struck in a perfectly ordinary aerobics class at the YMCA. The instructor had us doing some sort of weird bicycle-motion leg lifts at the end of the class, and I felt a little twinge in my left hip, in the front. It didn't seem like much at the time, but the next day I felt sore. Like a fool, I decided to shake it out by going for a little run. Big mistake. I felt OK during the run, but that night I was in a lot of pain, and the next morning I had to grab my knee and lift it up to get myself out of bed. I had strained a hip flexor muscle, or several of them, the ones that allow you to lift your knee. They also turn out to be really crucial to holding your torso in place when you're sitting. This led to yet another round of physical therapy, and a lot of frustrating time where I was reduced to swimming without kicking for my workouts. And I could only do that two or three times a week, or my shoulder would act up. This injury took about three months to get over, and like the shoulder, it's something I have to pay attention to even today. But it taught me to be patient with myself and my collagen, and to be creative in finding other workouts. Can't run? Swim without kicking. Lift some weights, see if the exercise bike is an option. Bide your time.

As soon as I could walk more or less normally again, I went ahead and bought the recumbent. It was the most money I had ever spent on anything but a car, but I really, really wanted to feel the wind in my hair again. Or at least the sweat under my bike helmet. The bike was pretty fun, too, in a dorky sort of way. It was one giant tube with the pedals way in the front, a little front wheel, and a cushy foam seat with a mesh back. The handlebars connected to the front wheel and came up at the sides of the seat. When I first tried to ride it, I felt like I was five years old and needed training wheels. When I got used to it, I reveled in the kicked back riding position and the unobstructed view of the scenery.

OK, status quo for a while. I kept working out, nursing all my achy parts, and watching my food intake. I made it under 200 pounds for the first time in about eight years, and I kept working. I ran a 10K race and got pretty close to ten-minute miles. I worked my way down to 195 for my wedding to that same long-limbed boyfriend. Nothing like a corset-tight wedding dress to inspire you to diet, right? In the weeks before the wedding I had nightmares about getting stuck in really tight waterslides, or staircases, or tunnels. Then I had this other dream that we were all going to do the wedding in elaborate Japanese costumes, à la "The Mikado." Nice, loose, flowing kimonos. Don't need no Sigmund Freud to tell me I was a little worried about that dress.

THE ROAD TO THE TRI

I FELL IN love with triathlon on July 20, 2001. It was a complete surprise to me, and probably to triathlon, too. If I thought of triathlon, I pictured whippet-thin, grim-faced automatons suffering through the 140 miles of Ironman Hawaii. Clearly I could never, ever do that. For one thing, I was still very far from lean, and, for another, that level of training and fitness and dedication was something I could never picture myself achieving.

But one spring evening at step aerobics, the stocky, middle-aged instructor announced that she was training for a triathlon, that she had finished dead last in her first one, and that she was determined not to be last next time. "Hmmm," I thought, having my first glimmer that people could participate in triathlon and still have body fat. Then in July, I went to watch my friend Russ competing in his first tri, a friendly, fuzzy little race called Tri For Fun. I saw him swim 400 yards, ride his bike for 13 miles, and run 3.1 miles. "Hey," I thought. "I could do that." Russ is pretty fast and lean, but he's a real human being, not an obsessed freak. He may have become an obsessed freak by now, but that's another story. "Sheesh," I exclaimed as he prepared for the start, "if I'd known these distances were so weeny, I'd have signed up, too!" Russ looked a little hurt. "It's a sprint distance," he responded. "It's not 'weeny.'" I was impolitic, but enthused. Next year, I thought, that'll be me.

In the fall I joined the Silicon Valley Triathlon Club (SVTC). I didn't really know where to start, but the Web site advised showing up for Tuesday night track workouts. OK. I started showing up. At my first workout, I felt completely blown out about two minutes into the warm-up. There were people there who didn't look like they were in that great shape, but they were clearly able to handle the warm-up. The warm-up was weird, too, running up and down the football field doing bizarre contortions called "high knees," "puddle jumpers," and "karaoke." The workout was intimidating, but the people weren't. I met a dude named Hans who wore smiley-face socks and claimed to be a distributor of rubber chickens. I didn't make it through that first workout. It was five repetitions of one thousand yards each. I was left behind in about the first two hundred yards, and it got worse from there. Eventually, after three painful reps, Gina, the nice assistant coach, took pity on me. "That's enough for your first time out," she said.

It took me weeks to learn that the nice assistant coach was actually Gina Kehr, a top pro triathlete who had finished eighth in the previous year's Ironman Hawaii. I immediately developed a schoolgirl case of hero worship, which I have not yet gotten over.

So I kept turning up for weekly humiliations at the club track workouts, and looked forward to the spring, when the races started. On December first, I joined the mad online stampede of hopeful entrants into Wildflower, the huge triathlon festival weekend that kicks off the season for the West Coast. I signed up for the mountain bike tri, a sprint distance race on May fifth. The clock was ticking. I didn't have a mountain bike, but I figured that for the short term I could borrow back the one I bequeathed to my brother after the hand therapist had offered his depressing prognosis.

What I wasn't sure of was whether I could ride a normal bike at all. I had gotten pretty comfortable on my recumbent bike, but I didn't know if I could subject my wrists and shoulder to the stress of a traditional upright bike. The recumbent community calls regular bikes "wedgies," but that wasn't the end I was worried about.

For the longer term, I needed a bike of my own, since I planned to do more triathlons if I could. I needed to be cautious about spending money, in case the grand experiment was all for naught. I headed to the Internet auction sites and started searching eBay. I didn't have a lot of work to do at my regular job, and this was a good way to kill time. (If any of my current bosses is reading this, I would never, ever surf the Internet at work if the company wasn't going down the toilet.) My dedication was rewarded. I saw a gleaming new, eleven-year-old bike of about the right size. The owner had gotten it as a present and literally never ridden it. It was made by Specialized, a very reputable company, and it had a swanky carbon-fiber frame, albeit an early version of this space-age technology. The components were good, my cycling friends told me, and it was probably a sweet deal. I sniped the auction and snuck in my winning bid of about $378 with mere seconds to spare.

Another chunk of money thrown at the local bike shop for adjustments, a comfy new saddle, new pedals, and a tune-up, and I was in business. My first ride was a ten-minute adventure, just to see if my hands would hold up. In tiny increments, I worked up to an hour on the bike. Things were looking good.

But then (there has to be a "but then," right?) I hurt my back later in the year while escaping a burning house in the middle of the night, and that put a damper on my training yet again. I couldn't run for about three months, and when I got back out on the road, I had to work back up into it, if not from square one, then at least from square three or so. I could barely do two miles, and it was only three months to race time. Fortunately in my first race, the run leg was only two miles, but I wanted to have a little cushion in my preparations. I had no training plan other than doing some swimming, biking, and running every week, and meeting up with other newbies from the tri club on weekends for longer rides or runs. So when the back got better, I did those things and waited for spring.

Spring came slowly for me that year—I was eager for Wildflower and the season. My tri club held a training camp weekend down at Lake San Antonio, the remote and rugged site of the Wildflower races. I was still in groveling awe of the people who were going out to ride the "long course" on their exotically engineered bikes, up and down fifty-six miles of hills with names like Nasty Grade, Heart Rate Hill, and Little Nasty. I was going to ride the ten miles of the mountain bike course, having recovered my off-road machine from my brother. I hadn't ridden off the pavement since 1997, but it worked out pretty well.

My really big worry about the whole race was: What the heck was I going to wear? Before you males scoff, "Oh, typical skirt," let me clue you in. I was worried about the swim and the run. The only sports bra burly enough to contain my "girls" when I run and keep them within the bounds of common decency is this armor-like contraption made by Enell. It is great for running, but it's not made of anything remotely like a bathing suit. So my big accomplishment of the weekend was swimming in the lake with the Enell and discovering that even when it was soaking wet, it still provided the Valkyrian firmness I required, without annoying chafing. You will learn that chafe-avoidance tactics are really big in the triathlon world—and the bigger you are, the more opportunities you have to learn about chafing.

Wildflower weekend finally arrived. Finally! After all the training, agonizing, reading, making checklists, and rehabbing injuries large and small, I loaded my gear and my husband in the car, and we went camping. This is the great thing about Wildflower. You've got thousands of athletes, from world-class pros to rank beginners, plus all the staff, volunteers, and spectators, crammed into the campgrounds of a Monterey County park. There's no hotel closer than an hour's drive. No fast food, no bike shop, nothing but the resort store by the lake. You have to ride your bike down a one-mile hill to get to the start, and after the race, you get to walk it back up again. The weather is usually scorching, the hills are insane, and the lines for the bathrooms stretch into the heat-shimmering horizon. It's an adventurous way to start any race season, and particularly inconvenient for launching yourself as a triathlete. Nevertheless, there we were. It's a custom among many triathletes and cyclists and other folks who suffer for fun to document their events in "race reports," so I got into the tradition with my very first race. You'll see more of these throughout the book.

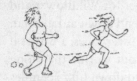

Deflowered at Wildflower

May 4, 2002
Mountain Bike Sprint Triathlon: 400-meter swim
| 10.2-mile bike | 2-mile run
Lake San Antonio, California

Wildflower, the Woodstock of triathlon. Second largest triathlon in the world. Nasty Grade, Heart Rate Hill, and dozens of other hills. Six thousand people. Legends of the sport: Scott Tinley, Steve Larson, Gina Kehr, Lori Bowden, Heather Fuhr, Becki Gibbs. Oh, and me. First triathlon ever, overweight by fifty pounds, coming off a tweaked back and a three-week "taper." [A period of reduced training before a big race, designed to rest the body and improve performance.]

I should have been scared. Slow runner, poor hill climber. Hills are hard on the back. Did I mention that there are hills at Wildflower? First open water swim, with the flailing limbs in the murky lake, with my new wetsuit. Is that wetsuit really the right size? My god, it's hard to get on. My first attempt at it, four days earlier, was a mixture of pathos and slapstick, with my husband Tim voicing a sincere concern that I could injure myself.

Maybe I shouldn't have been able to sleep the night before. What if my bike broke down? What if I swam off course and off toward King City? What if I came in last? What if I hurt my back and couldn't finish at all?

As it turned out, I was just happy. Happy to get my registration packet with its high-tech timing chip and silver swim cap. Delighted to put my race numbers on my bike, helmet, and belt. Pleased as punch to curl up in our tent on the freezing cold lumpy ground wearing five layers of clothing, a stocking cap, and gloves. And waking up at 5:45 on a foggy race morning to ride down Lynch Hill to the start? What could be better?

Great position in the transition area: last rack, halfway along. Easy to find, easy to get in and out. I racked my bike, laid out my stuff just as I had read about it, just as we practiced it, got my body marked—ooh, tickles!—wandered over to find Tim and watch the pros start. I tried to relax on the grass above the swim start. Didn't do so well. Popped up to watch my friend and inspiration, Russ, go off in his wave for the long course. Quick pit stop and off to the races.

The sun breaks out just as I head for my transition spot. Good omen? I met my rack mates, almost all first-timers, too. We shared our fears—is it really worth a wetsuit for four hundred meters? Is the water that cold? I rationalized that I am practicing for longer swims in colder water, so the wetsuit comes on. Also, if I don't wear the wetsuit, I'll be swimming in a loose tank top over my sports bra. Very unstylish. First the Bodyglide, then the PAM spray, so I'm slicker than a greased pig. Slow and patient, inching the suit up the legs, getting the wrinkles out, careful not to put a hole in the wetsuit.

OK, now it's 9:45 and the swim leg of the mountain bike race is starting. I'm almost to the gate and oops! Still got my hat on. Finally, my wave's about to go, we're warming up, the water feels perfect. Whoa! That was the horn! I start to swim, bumping bodies and elbowing my way through the water. I'm going pretty good until I bump something hard. It's one of the safety surfboards at the edge of the course. Hmm, not so good on the navigation. But I'm off again, relaxed, rolling, breathing, hardly kicking, saving my energy. Around the big orange buoy and I'm heading in, standing up, stumbling forward, I get the top half of my suit off and I'm jogging up to my bike. This is great!

A miracle! The bottom half of the wetsuit glides off over my greased limbs. My best friend Michelle is hanging over the fence, taking pictures. My bike shoes go on, my helmet strap clips, I'm heading for the bike exit. I feel fresh, I'm racing! I pass some people, even on hills. I lose a water bottle, but figure I'll survive. Now it's the sweet, fast downhill by the boat ramp, followed by the evil uphill that goes for the next two miles. I get good momentum, and the climb to the first loop turn is pretty painless, though for some reason I can't actually get a deep breath. A little adrenaline? "First lap right, second lap left!" the volunteers are screaming.

Now the fun downhill, and a fearless grab of a Gatorade bottle on my way to the second time up the two-mile hill. Bless the volunteers. Now I'm on the second climb and I still feel OK. Some people pass me, I pass some people. This is great! I remember to look around at the incredible view and thank volunteers whenever I have breath.

Dust in my face on the final stretch, and the short, steep Nasty Pimple before the sweet, sweet glide down Lynch Hill. Nobody's gonna pass me on this down-hill. Uh-uh, no way. Doff helmet, switch shoes, grab hat and race belt, and jog out. My legs are rubber, but there are people from the tri club cheering me on. Yay! Twenty minutes, more or less, and I'll be done. This is great!

The run course is all little rollers, up and down along the lake. Still trying to enjoy the scenery, but it's a lot easier to do so on the downhills. But there are people cheering for me, slow me, jogging along at my eleven-minute mile pace! Hit the turnaround and pick up a little momentum, but the last tiny rise before the finish just about kills me. I'm grimacing and gasping and pumping my legs to try and get up a hill that my grandma wouldn't notice on a bad day.

But the finish line is in sight, and there's Tim, and I hear cheers, so I pick it up as the beautiful, beautiful finish line draws near. I'm grinning. I think I've been grinning for the past hour and a half. Or day and a half. The fabulous volunteers are taking off my chip, handing me a wet towel and a medal? I get a medal? Me? This is great!

Water, fruit, and searching for Tim. He's there. He's so cool! I grab my Wildflower T-shirt and put it on over my sweaty race top cause I've earned it. A tri virgin no more. After months of training and reading and dreaming, it has happened: I am a triathlete, and Wildflower was perfect for my first time. Tough and rugged, gorgeous and leaving me wanting more. Much more.

We meet up with super-friend Michelle and watch Russ go out on the bike and come back in for his finish. I still feel like a wimpy slug compared to the long course heroes (and they're *all* heroes), but I also feel like a champion. I've got a gnarly blister on my toe, and my back's a little tender. But I've got endorphins to last for days, and I haven't had this much fun since my wedding.

So, two weeks until Uvas South Bay Triathlon—longer swim, longer ride, longer run. Can't wait.

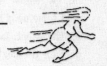

The Slow Fat Triathlete
Recommends

A FEW PRACTICAL TIPS TO SET YOU ON YOUR WAY

First of all, do you even want to be on your way? Is a triathlon something you're considering doing, or dreaming of doing, or are you reading this book from a strictly theoretical standpoint? If you do think you might want to, someday, dive in and do a tri, here are a couple of tips for reading the rest of the book:

1. Open Your Mind. Open up to the possibility that you can do this. Every time you catch yourself thinking, "Oh, this would just be too hard," or "I'm too old to do a triathlon," or "There's no way I could make the time to do this," stop and think, "Well, what if I could?" What if you are capable of it? What if you're not too old or too busy?

2. Think Long-Term. It took me about three years of getting gradually more fit before I was able to think that I would be fit enough to do a triathlon. Part of why I'm writing this book is to shorten that timeline for

you a little. But if you can't walk around the block today, you probably aren't ready for a triathlon twelve weeks from now. If you persist, though, you will get ready in your own good time.

3. Decide to Make It Fun. From my perspective, the best way to get something done is to define it as fun. If you want to do it, but you don't think it's going to be fun, why exactly do you want to do it? So as you're reading along, see if you can picture this whole wacky triathlon world as being fun for you.

4. Don't Worry about How You Look. Seriously. This is probably the most important point of this whole book, so I'm going to return to it over and over. If I had worried about looking fat and jiggly, or old and slow, every time I went out for a walk or a jog, I would never have done it. Before you read another word of this book, start implanting in your mind the thought that if you're doing something you like and something that's good for your body and mind, then how you look when you're doing it is the absolute least important thing in the world. Besides, you'll look fine. Nobody criticizes us as harshly as we criticize ourselves. Conversely, you could rationalize that even champion triathletes don't really look that sleek by the time they get done with the race. Haggard, sweating, sunburned, windburned, stringy-haired, and covered with salt stains—it's not a fashion show out there.

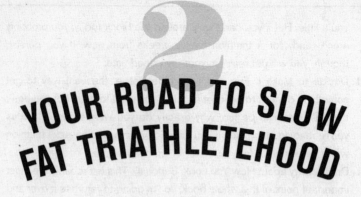

YOUR ROAD TO SLOW FAT TRIATHLETEHOOD

(OR FAST SKINNY TRIATHLETEHOOD, IF YOU INSIST)

So IN THE last chapter you read about my tottering first steps into triathlon, culminating with the wild mountain bike adventure at Wildflower weekend. I was so hooked, I couldn't wait for my next race and it was only two weeks away. Even though I injured myself yet again in the middle of my first season (more back pains) and had to skip a couple of races, I was still completely fired up to do another three races in the early fall, move up to Olympic distance races, and devour as much information about the sport as possible. And I did. The Olympic distance races were even more fun, and when the season was finally over I felt bereft. But I could always tell other people about how much fun I had.

SPREADING THE WORD

SINCE BECOMING A slow fat triathlete, I've turned into a tireless proselytizer for the sport, especially when it comes to people who are overweight or think of themselves as "non-athletes." When my training or racing comes up in conversation—and it does, frequently, because I can't shut up about it—I see this mix of incredulity and awe on people's faces. "You did *what*? But you're, um, kind of, um, *fat!*" I can also see their brains ticking away, calculating the odds of my being clinically insane. I can even see this reaction electronically in e-mails or message board posts. But almost every day, I get a post or an e-mail or a question from somebody who's contemplating maybe thinking about starting to train for a triathlon someday, but they don't know how to go about it.

So I spend time every week posting messages or e-mails to mostly overweight women, telling them that they can absolutely do a triathlon, that they can do far more than they imagine, and that they can start today. I tell them how I got started, and how heavy I was, and how I didn't have a bike, and maybe some of them have even done triathlons because someone told them they could.

WHY DO I CARE SO MUCH?

TRAINING AND RACING makes me feel just a little bit like Lance Armstrong (who started his athletic career as a teenage pro triathlete, by the way). I certainly don't have his freakish lung capacity, or the perfect length femur for cycling, or his body's ability to withstand physical stresses, or five yellow jerseys from the Tour de France. But when I'm training in the cold and rain or in the baking sun, grinding up a nasty hill, I usually hit a point where I'm completely in the moment. There's just the rhythm of my steps, or the sound of my arms moving through the water, or the endless circles of my pedal strokes. Every movement is an end in itself, every breath is the purpose of my life. It's all about breathing and going forward and breathing again. And I know that Lance has to do that, too.

It's also about gritty-sounding boot-camp nouns like dedication, commitment, perseverance, and sheer stubbornness. It's about sweating through every layer of your clothes, medicating your saddle sores, losing a toenail to a long run, learning to live with the burn of lactic acid in your body for longer than you could have believed possible. I never knew until triathlon that I could breathe so hard for so long that my rib muscles would hurt the next day. I think there are a lot of women around my age (just turned forty) and older who haven't necessarily had or taken the opportunity to challenge themselves to that degree. Fortunately a lot of other women have done amazingly hard, cool things athletically, and they're amazing role models. But sometimes those role models seem so lean and remote that it's hard to connect with them. I feel like a lot of people can connect with me.

Triathlon also provides me with an outlet for certain underlying geeky tendencies. I love to log my workouts, chart my race plans, calculate what percentage of women between the ages of thirty-five and thirty-nine came in ahead of me in all my races to date. I have a voracious appetite for information on anatomy, physiology, nutrition, and especially injury prevention. I love being my own science experiment. "Let's see, if I eat one banana twenty minutes before a workout, will I perform better than if I suck down a Clif gel thirty minutes into it?" I love the combination of analysis, planning, and preparation before a race or workout and pure action during the exercise itself.

Another thing that keeps me burrowing further and further into triathlon is that the tri community rocks. No other sport I've ever been involved with is as welcoming to newcomers as triathlon. At my tri club track workouts, Gina Kehr, a top-ten finisher in Ironman Hawaii, stands in the infield coaching the slowest, most exhausted folks around the track. People with eight thousand dollars worth of bicycle between their legs will stop and help you adjust the brakes on your four-hundred-dollar used beater. You can stand in the transition area and watch the fastest pro triathletes in the world setting up their towels and racking their bikes just a few feet away from your own spot. And the credo of every participant being a winner is more than just feel-good hot air; people live it. At a local series of races that I love, the race organizers make a point of bringing the last finisher up onto the festival stage for an enthusiastic ovation and the chance to say a few words about his or her race experience. It almost makes me want to be last.

It's not like being a fat person in a skinny sport is completely without tensions. There are plenty of times when I've felt like I didn't belong anywhere near a triathlon. This often happens when trying on tri clothes, when the biggest size women's race top they make only fits on my forearm. But it's pretty much always that way. If you're a large woman in America, your whole life is an opportunity to feel self-conscious, embarrassed, resentful, and *way* too big. You can hide in the corner or on the couch, you can go to therapy, or you can put on your Lycra bike shorts and get out there and move. So someone might drive by you and think, "My, what a tub." So the hell what? They're probably on their way back from Krispy Kreme anyhow. And if you're riding or running hard enough, you don't have time to care about what other people might be thinking. Besides, bike shorts, helmets, wetsuits, and goggles look dorky on everyone, especially if you wear them all at the same time.

WE ALL LOOK DORKY, AND LET'S NOT FORGET IT

TRIATHLON INCLUDES INNUMERABLE opportunities for low comedy, and I think that's absolutely critical to the overall experience. You learn about life. You learn about yourself. And a huge part of learning about yourself is being able to embrace your own ridiculousness. Yes, you can feel heroic as you dig down deep to get up the big hill or pass the person in front of you. You can feel the spiritual transcendence of being one with your body, communing with nature and your fellow triathletes.

But when you fall flat on your ass in the middle of transition because you can't get your cold, shaking legs out of your slippery wetsuit, it balances out the epic grandeur quite nicely. The drills we do to warm up for running look like mass practice for Monty Python's Silly Walks competition. We crash into each other trying to get on our bikes at the first transition. And we all pee in our wetsuits, don't let anyone tell ya different. And the contortions both men and women engage in so they can put anti-chafing creams on their various body parts—nobody looks anything but completely silly doing that. Nobody looks "good" when they're soaked with sweat and the Gatorade they spill on themselves during the run leg. I happen to think that shiny skin-tight Lycra is a fine fabric for all-day wear, but I know a lot of my girlfriends and my husband think we look, well . . . funny.

We look funny during our training, even funnier during our races, and our fears, neuroses, and pre-race nerves make us pretty funny, too. We worry about our fitness, about the weather, about the course layout, about our equipment, nutrition, sleep—it pretty much never ends. We're all a bunch of Woody Allens out there, right until the moment we step up to the line and hear the starter's horn. And then we go, ready or not, fat or thin, fast or slow.

What I'm really trying to say here (again) is that life is way too short and precious to worry about what other people think when you're out doing something. Self-consciousness is the enemy of fun. It's the enemy of feeling comfortable. It's the enemy of achievement. It's your enemy. Decide right now to banish self-consciousness from your journey to triathletehood. Don't worry about what you look like in Lycra, or whether your boobs jiggle when you run, or whether your beer belly gets in the way of your aerodynamic tuck on the bike. Remember, we all look dorky. And absolutely remember that we always think we look worse than we do. Believe that your body, like any body, was made to be moved, and that any body in motion is a glorious thing.

They say that nobody ever thinks on their deathbed, "Gee, I wish I had spent more time at the office." Yet I hear people say to me, "I'd love to do a triathlon, but I need to lose some weight first." Why wait? If you have any inkling of a longing to cross the finish line and raise your arms in triumph, just start now. Say to yourself, "My journey to the triathlon starts today." It starts with a single walk or jog, or a visit to the pool you haven't been to in years.

"BUT HOW DO I START?"

THE MOST IMPORTANT answer is: slowly. I'm not going to lay out detailed training plans because everyone has a different level of fitness and experience. The single biggest key to getting into an endurance sport is patience. If you've never run before, start by walking. If you can't walk around the block without getting pooped, work up to that first. Try a few minutes on an exercise bike, or a lap in the pool. Don't worry about how long it takes you. Be kind to yourself. You're taking your first baby steps in a new discipline. If you were coaching a baby to learn to walk, would you start out by dragging the little human on a five-mile run? No, you would not. And even if you tried, the experience would be so miserable that it would never be repeated. You'd injure the baby physically and emotionally. Be patient with your baby triathlete self. Your joints, ligaments, muscles, heart, lungs, and mind all need time and a gradually increasing workload in order to adapt to what you want them to do. If you don't give them that time and that slow buildup, you're going to get physically hurt and frustrated. And that's not fun.

I'll go into the nuts and bolts of training a little bit more in Chapter Four, so if you really want to talk about how exactly to swim, bike, and run to prepare yourself for triathlon, that's where to find that. What I want to talk about now is getting yourself ready to commit to a race.

FIND A RACE

I FIND THAT nothing sharpens my focus like a looming deadline. When I decided to get into triathlon, I knew that I wanted to do the first race of the upcoming season. I probably gave myself too much time to get prepared, given that I could already swim, bike, and run the distances I was planning. But on December 1, 2001, I entered the Wildflower Mountain Bike tri scheduled for the following May fifth. And when May came around, by God I was ready to roll.

So I strongly recommend picking a target race, with enough lead time so that you can train, but soon enough so that you feel the need to start your training now. Today. Or tomorrow if you need to get a pair of running shoes today. And do yourself a favor, right? Make your first race a sprint distance. Even if you're really fit and confident and all that (and if you are, why are you reading this particular book?), there's a lot to think about when you do your first race, so you should do a sprint and concentrate on logistics.

Get on the Web and enter "triathlon" and your local area into Google. If you don't have Web access, I have no idea how to advise you. Go get a computer and an e-mail account, or borrow a friend's, or use the public library. It's hard to do this sport without the Web and e-mail. There must be people who do it but I can't figure out how. I suppose you could go to a local running store or a pool or a bike store and ask the nice folks there about triathlons in the area. A lot of urban areas have a magazine called *CitySports* which lists tons of events.

Triathlon's really getting big in the US and internationally, so you should be able to find a race or two within striking distance. I Googled "triathlon peoria illinois" just now and got 474 results. You might have to drive a couple hours to get there, but you can choose from some cool-sounding races. The Iron Horse Triathlon, the TinMan, and Tri-Umph, for folks fifty-five and older. Hot Springs, Arkansas? Even more tri action. Laramie, Wyoming, boasts the Buffalo Triathlon in June. There's also a cool Web site called active.com, where you can search for races all over the country and often register online. OK, now you try. Got one? Good. Now sign up. You're going to do a triathlon.

FIND A CLUB

WHAT WILL OFTEN happen when you are looking for races is that you'll also come across the names of local triathlon clubs. This may be the best thing you'll ever find if you want your life to be transformed into a never-ending parade of track workouts, training rides, swim clinics, and social whirls. I found the Silicon Valley Triathlon Club this way, and this is one of the most amazing webs of people, resources, training opportunities, and fun that I have ever come across. I found out that SVTC had a "New to the Sport" program going and welcomed newbies with open arms. Not all clubs are like this, but from perusing the Internet at some length, it seems to me that most of them are. There are some clubs that are focused exclusively on the needs of fast, skinny people—and certainly those people do need a lot of special help—but by and large, the large, the slow, the inexperienced are encouraged to join in and get going.

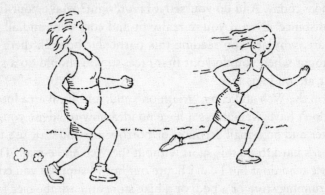

This doesn't mean that it will be easy to keep up with everyone when you first get going. It just means that people will smile and wave and say, "Great job!" as they lap you. This kind of support and encouragement can really make the difference between quitting on your second lap and hanging in there for another, oh, five minutes or so.

USA Triathlon, the governing body of most triathlons in the United States, has a list of affiliated clubs on its Web site. There are lots of triathlon clubs out there, though, that haven't gone through the process of affiliation, so if that list doesn't find you a local club, keep trying.

Clubs are fantastic sources of information about training, equipment, technique, races, places to run and ride, and other stuff. Plus you may get cool benefits like club discounts at stores or on race entries, and the all-important club logo gear. I treasured my royal blue SVTC logo socks until the heel wore out (see section on frivolous socks, Chapter 3), but the garish race wear in fabrics developed to keep astronauts warm, dry, and muscular for long space flights, ooh, that stuff continues to give me chills.

TRI FOR A GOOD CAUSE

ANOTHER WAY THAT a lot of people get into their first triathlon is through a noble effort to raise funds for a worthwhile medical cause.

The Leukemia & Lymphoma Society runs Team in Training (TNT), a purple-and-green-clad bunch that has single-handedly brought thousands of new triathletes to the sport and leads the pack by a large margin. In fact, I can't think of another organization that recruits as many new folks to the sport as TNT. (Astute readers will observe that the real acronym should be TIT, which I think would add a lot of humor to the undertaking, especially for the many women taking part.)

The way that TNT works is that you commit to raising some hefty amount of money for the cause, and in return you get access to free coached workouts, guaranteed entries in select races, discounted gear, and a vast support network around the country. TNT has such big contingents at some races that they have their own encampments and their own start times. They specialize in getting people from couch potato to triathlete status, so they really are a good option for a lot of novices. If you feel that you're particularly slow and out of shape, you are likely to find company at the TNT group workouts in your area, and that can be a fine thing.

No matter how you enter the world of triathlon, on your own, through a club, through Team in Training or another fundraising group, enjoy yourself, enjoy your training, and take a lot of pride in what you're doing.

WHAT ARE YOU WAITING FOR?

ARE YOU FEELING at all excited about this? Are you tempted to schedule your upcoming race season, drag the old bike out, head over to the pool at the Y? Or are you experiencing the queasy negativity of self-consciousness? Of self-doubt? Are you thinking, "That's probably fun, but it's not something I could do. I'm too fat/old/injured/busy/apathetic to go through with it. Besides, people will see my body in shorts and it will be on the evening news that my body differs significantly from the US-MTV-certified ideal." Or are you thinking, "Man, this chick is twisted. Why on earth would anyone even want to make themselves uncomfortable for hours on end for a T-shirt and a couple of free Clif Bars?" If the latter, congratulations, you have passed the intelligence test hidden in the first two chapters of this book. Don't worry about actually doing any of the stuff I'm writing about. You probably have the kind of serene, Zen-like personality that assures you that you have nothing to prove to yourself or others. It's the rest of us restless, dissatisfied, neurotic seekers that feel the need to show we can do it. And if you feel that need at all, but you are worried about your readiness to do it, that's all the more reason why you should just do it.

YOUR COMPETITIVE FIRE—BLESSING OR CURSE?

I WAS JOGGING along this morning with Dave, another slow fat triathlete from my club, and he was explaining to me that he was working through a crisis of motivation after completing his first half-Ironman distance triathlon. He had worked hard all winter, spring, and summer, had dropped a lot of weight and improved his endurance tremendously. But his time in the race was slower than he had been shooting for, and he felt his performance compared unfavorably to several other club members whom he thought should have been around his level. I think he was a little bummed that a sixty-two-year-old woman had about the same bike and run times as he did. Never mind that she's been doing it a long time, that she's qualified for the World Championships in her age group, or any of that. He felt slow and he was bummed. So instead of reveling in his fantastic accomplishment—being a dude in his forties who took only ten months or so to get in good enough shape to swim 1.2 miles, bike 56, and run a half-marathon in the hot August sun—he was beating himself up for still being slow and fat.

When Dave started sharing his feelings with fellow triathletes of all levels, they supported him like good friends. They praised his dedication, his determination, and the fact that he finished the race. They pointed out how far he had come in such a short time. And Dave, being an intelligent kind of guy, started to realize that he had defined his goals in such a way that it was depriving him of fun. He was feeling like a failure because he wasn't fast, rather than feeling like an incredible success story for being a disciplined, enthusiastic, competent triathlete who also volunteers for the club in all kinds of ways and draws people to him with his warmth and energy. So he was in the process of switching gears, starting to swap the "no pain, no gain" mentality for one that awards maximum points for effort, fun, and improvement, and de-emphasizes where he crosses the line in relation to other people. And it seemed to me that he was starting to have more fun.

I was pretty stoked to hear Dave's story, illustrating as it does that the mental pitfalls and rewards of triathlon are just as intense and significant as the physical aspects. For my money, this sport is demanding enough, without putting extra pressure on myself to measure up to someone else's standards. I can only do what I can do. When I'm training, I don't mind if someone else drops me on the road or on the track. I have to just measure my own efforts, figure out what kind of intensity I need to put into a given workout, and let the rest of the chips fall where they may. If I had started out being bummed out every time I was left behind in a workout, I probably would never have gotten to my first race.

Having said all that, I also admit that I'm massively competitive when I get into a race situation, mostly with myself and my past performances. I have goals for myself for each phase of the race and I really want to meet them. I also fight like hell to pass people on the bike and avoid being passed on the run. When I'm running, I pick people up ahead of me who look like they're not going too fast, and I concentrate on reeling them in slowly but surely. I want to feel completely spent at the end of the race and wouldn't be satisfied with anything else. I also compare my results to other people in my age group, to the field in general, how I did in my last race, and to my goals at the beginning of the season. I think for me the key to having goals and racing against other people is to make the goals realistic and to race the right people. I know I'm not going to run six-minute miles in a race, but it is realistic for me to shoot for nine-minute-fifteen-second miles after two years of training. I know I can't catch the top women in my age group, but it's for sure I can catch that woman up ahead who's having a slow day on the bike.

But I also concentrate a lot on having fun. The race is the big payoff for all the training, right? This is where you have to put your faith in the work you've done and just let it hang out on the road. I always make a point when I race of looking around at the scenery, thanking the volunteers, and reminding myself that it's a fantastic privilege to be able to do a race at all. I think back on my injured, obese, frustrated past, and I revel in the joy of being able to move freely and work my body hard. I may never win a race or even come close, but when I can feel the joy of movement and experience the beauty of the world by racing through it with my eyes wide open, that's a victory every time.

For me, what makes triathlon so addictive and fun is finding this balance for myself between achievement and process. An actor isn't going to want to be an actor if he doesn't have a strong affinity for the whole process of putting a show up, from the first reading of lines to getting the technical elements together to the endless hours of rehearsal. But of course the rush of performance, being on stage and showing the results of all that effort, is a peak experience. Same with triathlon for me. I would never get to the race if I didn't enjoy the whole journey of training, slowly building my endurance, working on strength and speed, comparing notes with my friends, doing that long Saturday ride or the Tuesday night track workout. The high of the race, though, is just incomparable.

As you get moving on this journey, keep looking for your own balance. What's going to make this fun for you? Don't get so caught up in numbers and hours of training that you lose sight of the joy of moving. Think of yourself as a lucky, lucky kid, who gets to spend time in the pool, then riding around on your bike, then running around the hills and woods in the neighborhood. What could be better?

SO IT'S A GO, RIGHT?

ALL RIGHTY THEN! Contrary to your own best judgment, you sign up for a race. Maybe you even find a nice group of people to egg you on as you join them in their crazed delusions of what constitutes fun. Maybe you decide that your endeavor will largely be a solitary one. However you start, you need to get some gear, and you need to do some training. If you can just get off the couch and go do a tri of any distance, then put down this book, for god's sake, and go do it! Why are you wasting time reading on a beautiful day? Give this book to your mom and have her sign up for a race with you. But if you know as little about training and equipment as I did starting out, by all means read on.

And in case you were wondering how my race career progressed, here's a little something for ya. My first Olympic distance race was really a great mix for me of the joy and adrenaline and effort of the race day, and maybe this race report will capture a small part of that.

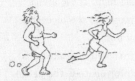

Stepping Up

September 29, 2002
Sentinel Triathlon(Olympic Distance): 1.5K swim | 40K bike | 10K run
Santa Cruz, California

Not that I'm a veteran triathlete, but I had three races under my belt by July of this year, and in my hubris I felt that I needed to move up from the sprint distance. You barely have time to get wet, cold, dizzy, chafed, exhausted, sunburned, dehydrated, cramped, and blistered and it's all over. Where's the fun in that?

My Oly distance debut was originally planned for Folsom in early August, but I bowed out with nagging hip/back stuff. So it came to pass that the Santa Cruz Sentinel (named for the local paper that sponsors it) was my first time to step up in distance. And of course I hadn't really had much injury-free time to train for the run. But at least I had been running. Or jogging. Getting cheerfully humiliated at track workouts three weeks in a row. That had to count for something.

Every race brings its own special irrational fear. My first race it was the hills. The second race it was the long run. The third it was the very very early wake up call. This time it was the looming threat of closing the course. The Sentinel folks said they would *close* the course at 11:45. I taxed my mathematical abilities to determine that if my wave started at 8:20 (the old ladies over thirty-five always go last, grrrrrr), I would have to finish in 3:25 or less to avoid the humiliation of stumbling in after the banners and balloons were long gone, not to mention the fruit and bagels. This was freaking me out. I didn't think I could do it in under 3:30. I thought forty-five minutes for the swim, maybe 1:40 for the bike, and 1:06 at best for the 10K run. Add in the transition times and I was clearly not going to make it. Especially with the sore shoulder sustained two weeks ago at Pacific Grove.

I slept poorly the night before, restless on the flocked surface of my Inflatabed, trying not to wake up Russ and Michelle, by whose goodness I was camped on the floor of the Best Western Santa Cruz. But the alarm went off as planned. The wheels were set in motion. I was just going to have to do what I could.

Dawn crept up on us as we arranged our complex array of gear in our cramped little transition area. It was clear and cold, and the chatter among the competitors focused on water temperature. We ambled down the hill to the beach and across the sands to the lifeguard tower at the start. "Ohmygod!" Michelle gasped, "look at the waves!" I scoffed like a native—"Ahhh, ankle high. Those aren't waves." Of course by the time I was ready to go in and warm up, the biggest set of the morning was breaking at heights far exceeding my own.

But I'm a native, so I waded in and dived under the first wall of white surf I encountered, holding onto my goggles with one hand. Unfortunately, the petite Asian woman in front of me did not know the dive-under technique. She was tossed around like a beach ball and bounced firmly onto my sore shoulder. This was discouraging. Good thing she was petite. I also noticed that the suspended sand in the water made a nice abrasive layer under my wetsuit. How did that even get *in* there? Oh, and the water was in fact cold.

I shuffled up onto the beach and met up with my husband Tim to exchange affectionate nuzzles. The race organizers had laid on actual bagpipers to make the moments before the start particularly stirring, and the first wave went off to the sound of actual guns fired by actual hairy men in kilts. By my wave, I was prepared for the godawful bang and I sprinted down the sand towards the water, diving in amid a flurry of arms and legs. I worked on keeping my stroke strong and controlled, and I noticed I was floating so high in the salt water that there was really no point in kicking my legs at all. So I streamlined my feet, rotated my body from side to side, and swam and swam and swam. Approaching the end of the pier, I heard strange honking noises. I rolled to my right and saw six massive sea lions basking in the early morning sun among the underpinnings of the pier. Aren't they supposed to be aggressive and territorial? I hoped they didn't perceive this odd aquatic procession as a threat.

At last the beach came into view and I staggered into an upright position, narrowly missing being tackled from behind by a hefty wave. Checked the watch—thirty-two minutes and forty seconds? No way! I'm way ahead of schedule here, like thirteen minutes ahead. Tim yelled and waved and took pictures as I lurched across the beach and up to the transition. Michelle yelled and waved and took pics a little further on, then she made a dash around to a spot just outside my rack. We had a nice little chat as I transformed myself from a neoprene super-hero to a soggy cyclist and headed out.

California Highway One up to Davenport is incredibly scenic. Rolling fields of brussels sprouts, golden hills covered with oak and cypress, cliffs dropping off to isolated sandy coves. The sun was shining and I was spinning my gears at a pretty good clip. The road undulated over the terrain in such a way that I could tuck over my bars and pick up serious speed on the downhills, getting enough momentum that I could coast halfway up the next hill. Cruising! I had to keep reminding myself not to go too hard on the bike. I figured I had to average fifteen miles per hour to get back in time to do the run—but I still had to have legs to do the run with. But I was having such a darn fine time going fast and I felt strong, so I just let it fly and made sure I didn't get too blown out on the uphills.

Amazingly, I was back at the transition after just an hour and twenty-two minutes, eighteen minutes ahead of pace. I had averaged eighteen miles per hour on the bike. I could walk the run leg now if I had to. And it was certainly tempting. After all, I'd already had two hard workouts this morning and it was just after 10 A.M. Michelle spotted me at the transition and said, "That was *fast!*" I felt pretty fast, yup. Another gulp of Cytomax, another energy gel in the pocket, and I was away again.

I will not make a secret of it: Running is hard for me. I feel the jarring impact of the pavement at every step. I feel my (possibly crappy) knee cartilage fraying as I trot along. My flabby bits bounce, my back feels unnaturally tight, and people pass me at an alarming rate. That's on a good day. Now add in the first two legs of a tri and I'm just not loving it. This is where the suffering starts.

But I tried to love it. I want to get better, really I do. So I waved again to Tim, moved my rubbery legs along, trying to keep my breathing regular and my feet turning over quickly. I worked on enjoying the cliffs and the surfers and the waves and the people with big furry dogs and on not being discouraged when I was passed by the very people I had passed convincingly on the bike. There were lines of runners coming back already from the midpoint; in fact, the winners had already crossed the line by the time I started running.

I had planned to take little walk breaks in the race, just to give my legs a little recovery time. I was in the middle of one of those when Russ passed me with a high five. "You OK?" he called out. "Great!" I said. Of course I had only run a mile at the time. During another walk break, I called out to a volunteer on the course, "This is part of my strategy!" I felt it was important that this complete stranger know I was walking by choice, not necessity. He laughed in a kindly way.

Finally the turnaround point at 3.1 miles, two cups of cold water, and back along the same cliff path to the finish. It was just unimaginably far away. The lighthouse shimmering in the haze could have been in Cameroon as far as I was concerned. And how far was it from the lighthouse to the finish? Half a mile? If I thought about the distance I would get very depressed. Except that I was still running, and I knew I was going to make it to the finish one way or the other, and they weren't going to close the course on me unless I suddenly just fell down and couldn't move a limb.

Around the time I reached the lighthouse, falling down began to seem like an attractive option. I was consciously exerting the muscles of my ribcage to suck in more air, and I stumbled a couple of times on perfectly flat ground. My smile had turned into a grimace, and once again the voice of cycling commentator supreme, Paul Sherwen, ran through my head: "And right now, Phil, every muscle in her body is screaming for her to stop but she has to keep it up for just a little while longer yet." OK, who moved the freakin' finish line?

Oh, finally, finally, I could see it. And right about the same time, a woman came up onto my shoulder. She had passed me at about mile four, but I had caught her at the lighthouse and I was darned if she was going to pass me again. I put on my "kick" and "sprinted" to the finish, which made me want to puke as soon as I had crossed the line. I gasped for air and checked my watch. 3:09? Well, that's simply not possible, I thought to myself, and I looked again. It still said 3:09, plus a few seconds 'cause I had forgotten to push the stop button. I ran 6.2 miles in sixty-six minutes, which is about what I ran for my last 10K in March—without that swimmy-swimmy bikey-bikey thing beforehand. Yeah, it's slow, but for me it wasn't bad.

And then the rest was a warm pleasant blur of hugging and grinning and photos and bananas and packing up sodden gear at a very slow pace, until I came slowly to my senses in a booth in Denny's, staring into the barrel of a Grand Slam Slugger breakfast that was indescribably huge and tasty. Three hours plus, now that's a decent amount of pleasure/pain/pleasure/pain/pleasure. Next up— Treasure Island Triathlon. Swimming in the San Francisco Bay in November. Nothing to fear in that race, surely?

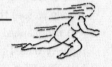

The Slow Fat Triathlete
Recommends

Cool! You're still with me. Here's my relentlessly practical, neatly-bulleted box o' tips to keep you on the road to your first race:

1. Abandon Self-Consciousness. I just can't say this enough: Self-consciousness is your worst enemy. I know I wrote about it just a few pages ago, but it is after all the most important point I have to make in this book, so I'll just keep saying it. Absolutely nothing good ever comes of worrying what other people think of you when you're doing something that you want to do, that's fun and legal, and that's actually good for you.

2. Be Real. Don't sign up for the World's Toughest Half-Ironman for your first race. Find something that looks like it's easy to get to and a pretty realistic goal for distance and terrain. The first race you do should leave you feeling like, "Man, that wasn't so hard! Let's do another one!"

not like, "Oooooohhhhhh my goooodddd, I barely survived that and I will now have to take to the couch for three weeks."

3. Use the Web. You can find out pretty much everything about triathlon by judicious use of the Internet. You can find out where the races are, sign up online, find a triathlon club, get beginners' training plans, learn what's what and who's who in the sport, get tons of nutritional and psychological advice, and generally waste a ton of time. If you have a boring cube job, just start Googling.

4. Who Are You, Anyway? Some people really need the social aspect of getting together and training with other people, feeling the warm glow of grouphood. Others really just want to make their plans and do their thing, on their own, without a club or a masters swim team or a weekly group bike ride. If the idea of joining a club makes you break out in a cold sweat, you don't have to. If you know you'll never ever get up and swim in the morning unless there's someone waiting for you at the pool, then look into the masters swim or recruit a training buddy. Figure out what style suits you as you start out. It might change later, but do what you're comfortable with right now.

3

IT'S REALLY NOT ABOUT THE BIKE

OBSERVATIONS ON EQUIPMENT—
ESSENTIAL, INESSENTIAL, AND FUN

THE INCOMPARABLE LANCE ARMSTRONG, the greatest and most famous cyclist America has yet produced, called his first book *It's Not about the Bike*. Lance, five-time Tour de France victor and survivor of extremely aggressive metastasized cancer, has unbreakable will, unmatched resiliency of body and spirit. Physically he's ideally suited for the rigors of bicycle racing, and his training incorporates the most advanced technology available. His incredible story of surviving and conquering against all odds really isn't about the bike. At the same time, if he didn't have a bike, that whole Tour de France thing wouldn't be happening.

So as you venture into the wacky world of multisport (insider jargon for "triathlon and its related offshoots"), you do need a little equipment. What I want to do in this chapter is break down the equipment into three basic categories, starting with the essentials you absolutely have to have to get to the starting line. Then we'll talk about stuff you can toss your hard-earned cash at if you think you might end up getting more seriously into this pastime. And then there are the frills—fur-lined saddle covers, carbon-fiber crank arms, and titanium bike gloves, that sort of thing. Ah—gotcha! There's no such thing as titanium bike gloves. I haven't seen the fur-lined saddle covers yet either, but the carbon-fiber pedal cranks are for real. Needless to say, the free market offers a dizzying array of goodies you can buy that might make your races or training easier, or just make you look like a person with way more bucks than brains.

IT'S NOT TOTALLY ABOUT THE BUCKS

YOU CAN SPEND a ton of money getting into this sport. You can easily drop three thousand dollars or more on a nice bike, five hundred dollars on a state-of-the-art wetsuit, two hundred dollars on your bike shoes, another one hundred fifty dollars on the helmet. But whoa! Take a cleansing breath. Don't throw this book away in disgust, cursing the elitist and expensive nature of triathlon. You can and should get started for way less money. Sometimes, though, an extra thirty dollars on a gadget is actually a great investment in your time or comfort. It's a tricky path to negotiate, so hold my hand and don't wander away, right?

This chapter is divided up into three main categories. Bare Essentials, Inessentials, and Fun Stuff. My definition of Bare Essentials is whatever you would absolutely need to complete your first race, which is probably a sprint distance. If I've seen people do without it in a race, it won't be on the bare essentials list. My second category, Inessentials, includes things that can make your training or racing more comfortable and/or more efficient, but you can get along without them if you are on a budget, have a minimalist approach, or don't think you're ever going to do more than one race. Finally, Fun Stuff is just that. It's great to find it in your Christmas stocking, but you really don't need it even for a whole season of triathlon. Let's take each category in the time-honored order of the triathlon events: swim, bike, run.

BARE ESSENTIALS:
DON'T LEAVE HOME WITHOUT THEM

THE SWIM: BARE ESSENTIALS

1. Swimsuit
2. Goggles
3. Wetsuit, if you are going to swim in any water colder than about 65 degrees

Swimsuit

The swimsuit seems pretty self-explanatory, yah? Basically it is. Hopefully you already have something you can swim in. If you don't, the two things you want to look for are durability and that snug, body-hugging fit. Guys, if you swim in your baggy board shorts, you're going to be working a lot harder than you need to, because the water resistance against those shorts is pretty significant. Suck it up: Buy a Speedo. Who cares if your girlfriend laughs at you? Females, forget the ruffled swim dress. In the water, streamlined is good. Ruffles are bad. If you're at a size where regular women's swimsuits seem like a cruel joke, check out www.junonia.com for a great variety of bathing suits and other exercise wear sized for the generously proportioned. When I started off in the pool, Junonia was my lifesaver. A suit that snugly contained my rather sizeable breast matter was really, really hard to find. Thanks, Junonia.

The suit should be pretty durable because you'll probably be putting in some pool time, and cheap suits just fall apart with that repeated exposure to chlorine and sun. Even some pretty expensive suits fall apart, too, so if you're buying one, quiz the sales guy about the expected life span of the offending garment. And if it does fall apart, buy another one.

Forget what I said above. You are going to end up spending a boatload of money on this sport.

Goggles

Swim goggles are pretty easy to deal with, and cheap, too. The key is trying them on to make sure they fit you. And don't be shy about doing this in the sporting goods store. They're all packed up in those annoying and impenetrable plastic bubbles, sure, but you can open those with minimal tools, and some progressive stores even have trays of samples you can try on. Press them up on your eyes and see if you get suction. They should stay on your face without the elastic. If they don't, they'll leak. One irritating fit issue with goggles is that a lot of them are designed with molded nose pieces, so that if you have a particularly broad or narrow bridge to your schnozz, it can be difficult to get a pair that do fit. Some brands still make goggles with adjustable nose pieces, so those can be a good option. When you do find the right combination of nose width and eyepiece size, get a couple or three pairs while you're at it. The lenses get scratched up in your gym bag, and the elastic eventually wears out and snaps, painfully, on your ear, right when you are about to start a swim. Plus, thanks to the inexorable grind of "progress," you may never be able to find that perfect model again.

Wetsuit

If you live in Florida or some other halcyon place where the water is always toasty warm, you can skip this part about the wetsuit. The rest of you, gather round. If the water you plan to race in is going to be seventy degrees or warmer, you don't have to worry about the wetsuit if you don't want to. There are some advantages to wearing one, but it's not essential if the water's not cold. Wetsuits are good because:

1. You float better in a wetsuit. The buoyant Neoprene acts like an all-over life preserver. You float high and bob around like a cork. This can make you feel a lot more secure in the water, especially helpful if you're not a confident swimmer.

2. You swim a little faster in a wetsuit. In general, the slower you are at swimming, the more you benefit from the wetsuit. Mostly it's the additional flotation. Since less of your body mass is below the surface of the water, there's less drag on your body and you go faster for the same amount of effort. It's not going to turn you from a manatee into an Olympian, but it can shave a couple of minutes off your time over a fifteen-hundred meter swim.

3. You feel like a superhero in a wetsuit. There's something about pulling that sleek, black Neoprene costume on that makes you feel like an aquatic being with special powers. The super-stretchy material compresses some of your bulgier bits and makes you feel strong. Add your goggles and the swim cap the race organizers provide, and the effect is complete. You are AquaTriWoman! You are FrogTriGuy! You swim like a shark, you breathe through your gills, the water is your native element!

4. You look funnier in a wetsuit. All the effects in point number 3 above are true. However, it is at least equally true that you look like a total dork. You're covered in rubber, for crying out loud! In addition, the contortions you go through in order to get into and out of the wetsuit on race day are absolutely rife with low comedy. It's the Three Stooges meets The Man From Atlantis, minus Patrick Duffy. "What the hell," I hear you ask, "is the advantage in looking like a dork?" There are two, mainly. One is that you take yourself less seriously that way. (More on this later.) The other is that spectators have a good time laughing at your maneuvers. This helps to grow the sport of triathlon.

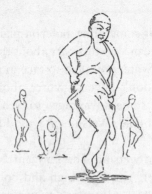

If the water you'll be swimming in is cold—and my beloved Northern California oceans are a prime example of cold waters for triathlon— then you really will need a wetsuit to go swimming. Hypothermia is no joke. Of course, I carry enough subcutaneous fat that it provides a lot of insulation from the cold. I call it my internal wetsuit. But I still put on my external wetsuit for ocean swims.

Don't stress too much about buying a wetsuit if you're only planning to try a race or two and see how you like it. If there is cold water in your area, chances are there's a place around where you can rent one. There are wetsuits made specifically for triathlon and open water swimming, which are harder to find as rentals. But you can definitely swim in a surfing or rafting or other kind of wetsuit. I see it all the time. The main features a tri wetsuit offers are extra-flexible material around the shoulders and a smooth exterior with minimal seams for decreased drag in the water. They're also super-stretchy, so they fit your body more tightly. For the slow fat triathlete, this is not always a great thing aesthetically speaking, but it helps make you more efficient in the water. The less water you're carrying around between your body and the inside of the suit, the better. The triathlon wetsuits are also the ones that offer the best superhero effects, described above. But my main point is—*don't* let wetsuit-related frugality keep you from doing a cool race. You can rent a wetsuit that will work and won't break the bank.

If you are interested in breaking the bank, or you already know you love triathlon so much that you must have your own tri-specific superhero wetsuit right away, by all means go for it. I bought mine before my first race, partly because I was concerned about finding a rental large enough to fit me, and also because I was convinced I was going to do enough races to make it worthwhile. When you go looking for a wetsuit, you should probably not do as I did (see sidebar on the next page). Instead, you should seek out a store that sells tri wetsuits and try a bunch on to see what fits you best. The different brands have different cuts and fit very differently.

How I Bought My Wetsuit:
A Cautionary Tale

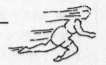

It was three weeks before my first triathlon. I had gone down to Lake San Antonio and done a little swim dressed in my finest nylon sports bra, tank top, and tri-shorts, and *dang!* It was cold. I needed Neoprene protection, prontissimo. I checked out rentals, but I figured I was going to be doing this thing for at least one season, so I started researching the different makers. Orca, Ironman, Quintana Roo, T1, Aquaman: The very names gave off a cold, crisp aroma of aquatic heroism.

A couple of things were immediately obvious, though. These wetsuits were pricey and they were constructed for stick figures. Checking out the sizing for Orca, I determined that, ideally, I should be about 6'5" to get a suit that would accommodate my body weight. But I read encouraging online posts about how stretchy the material was, and how people of stature not too different from my own were able to fit into them.

It was time for eBay. I spent a couple of hours over scattered days looking for the brand names that I wanted and finally found a floor demo Orca Speedsuit, size ten, for about sixty-five dollars off retail. Score! I jumped at it, clicked the "buy it now" icon, and anxiously awaited its arrival. I was a little nervous, but I had already discovered a booming classified market on various tri Web sites, and I figured I could sell it off to some other sucker.

When the wonderful package arrived, I tore into it like a kid at Christmas. It was beautiful. Sleek and black, with speedy-looking graphics reminiscent of mighty killer whales, it seemed to leap out of the box of its own power. "Look, honey! Isn't this cool?" I shrieked. I started to try it on right there in the living room. Immediately the wetsuit changed from a sleek, efficient killer whale to a sticky, all-engulfing monster from a cheesy science fiction movie. *Slow Fat Triathlete Meets the Pantyhose From Hell.*

I got my feet into the legs and embarked on a sweaty wrestling match, wherein the monster continually thwarted my efforts to insinuate my legs into the constrictive casings. I gave a yank to get the suit to inch up over my sturdy thighs, and wow! Look at that. I put a hole in it with my fingernail. I slumped to the floor, cursing. "Um, Jayne . . . don't injure yourself," Tim said anxiously. The worst was over though. Once I got the thing up and over my butt, the top half went on with only about half the effort. It was on!

Still, I couldn't really imagine how this process was going to help me be faster, either in the water or anywhere else. It had taken me about a half hour to get the thing on, it seemed like. Getting it off was easier, but not much. I was exhausted and dispirited, and now I had to find a way to fix the half-inch tear I had put in my brand new toy. This turned out to be pretty easy, using some weird black goo from the dive shop.

When it came to the race, I had been instructed in the fine art of applying PAM to pretty much every surface of my body to help the suit slide on and off. Yes, PAM. Non-stick cooking spray. I also had a stick of an anti-sticking, anti-chafing substance lubriciously called Bodyglide. I covered myself with both, to the point where I couldn't grasp the wetsuit because my hands were so slippery.

So here's what not to do, which I did:

1. Don't buy a wetsuit you haven't tried on. If you try on some and determine that you need an Orca size nine, then you can buy it online or used or for some crazy deal. Of course, trying them on in the store risks public humiliation, but they will at least have a little room for you to change in.

2. Don't tear your wetsuit when you put it on. Trim down your fingernails, and don't ever grab at the fragile Neoprene with your nails. Use the pads of your fingers, and be patient.

3. Whatever you do, don't try the wetsuit on for the first time in front of your significant other. Tim worried about me until after my first race was done, convinced I was going to sprain my greater medial anterior thingie or do other serious damage.

4. Don't put so much PAM on your body that you look like a Thanksgiving turkey greased for the oven. Apply judiciously—ankles, calves, thighs, shoulders—and have a towel handy to wipe your hands. Beyond a certain point, patience is more effective than lube.

THE BIKE: BARE ESSENTIALS

1. Bike
2. Helmet
3. Pump
4. Puncture repair

Bicycle

The bike is the arena where you can get seriously carried away with gear. The bikes themselves are so beautiful: gleaming, finely-wrought machines redolent of both tradition and cutting-edge technology. They will seduce you from their racks, insinuating voluptuous thoughts into your mind. "I will make you faster, lighter, more powerful, more stable. Buy me and you will be great." Do *not* listen to their siren song! Don't even take your wallet to the bike store if you're shopping around. You have to figure out what you need, what you want, and what you can afford, and then go nuts—oops, I mean make a rational decision. And I haven't even talked yet about all the wonderful accessories you can buy for your new pet.

If you already have a bike, great. You're set. Seriously. You can do your first tri or first five tri's on that old beater. Vintage beach cruiser? Bring it on. Citified "hybrid" bike? Even better. Mountain bike that hasn't been out of the garage in five years? Sweet. You don't need a fancy road bike to get started. If it has two wheels and working brakes, you can ride it in most any sprint-distance race. You can pedal *anything* for twelve miles or so. If you don't have a bike and money's tight, you can buy used. I'm not the total queen of eBay, but I did score my road bike there, and I've seen lots of good deals. A lot of people don't have the high tolerance for risk required to buy a bike sight unseen from a complete stranger, but if you have a bargain-hunting mentality and the willingness to turn around and resell your bike if it doesn't work out, this can be a great way to go.

I know there are a lot of new and about-to-be triathletes out there, though, who would like nothing better than to justify the purchase of a gleaming new piece of velocipedic machinery to go with their new hobby. We call you "yuppies." And god bless you all, because you're keeping the triathlon industry booming. So here are a couple of things to think about if you're going to hit the bike shops.

Figure out what you need for the kind of riding you're going to do. For most beginning triathletes, an entry-level road bike from a reputable manufacturer will be plenty good. Trek, Giant, Fuji, Cannondale all make reliable bikes that are widely available. A brand called Cervélo has a pretty sweet getting-started road bike for a good price, too. Terry Precision Bicycles makes bikes especially for women's proportions, which can solve a lot of problems for a lot of women. If you live in a really hilly area like I do, get a bike with a triple chain ring in front. The smallest chain ring, or "granny gear" to snobby road cyclists, can really help you get up those hills when they kick up to awe-inspiring gradients. Don't be like me. I bought a double chain ring and have been suffering up the hills ever since. Especially if you're heavy, go for the triple. You'll be so glad you did.

And you don't have to buy a road bike. You really don't. I see plenty of people out on the roads, racing in triathlons on mountain bikes or commuter bikes. If you only want one bike and you're going to spend most of your time on it going back and forth to the café for lattes, you may decide a commuter or "hybrid" bike with a more upright pedaling position and a nice cushy seat is the way to go. My attitude is that I weigh enough on my own, so I want my bike to be pretty light.

Find a good bike shop. I would recommend doing this by finding out where the folks in the local tri club or cycling club go for their tune-ups. Even if you don't buy your bike from them, a well-informed, helpful staff and a kick-ass service department are treasures to be cherished. They can help you get your bike adjusted to make your life much easier, you more comfortable, and your bike safer for you to ride. They can advise you on what you really need as opposed to what you might want or think you need.

Don't worry too much about the frame material or specs or all the technical aspects unless you like to geek out over that stuff. Ride the bike around as much as the shop will let you, and go with what feels good. Don't buy a bike that's not comfortable.

If you're going to actually buy a bike, you will probably be encouraged to buy special cycling shoes and "clipless" pedals. If you're already a cyclist, you know that clipless pedals are a little bit of a misnomer. They do attach your shoes to the pedals in a process we still call "clipping in," but without a big old-fashioned metal toe clip that comes up over your shoe and gets cinched down with a strap to the point of toe numbness. Instead, clipless pedals use a binding to attach to a cleat on the sole of your shoes. The systems vary, but basically you step onto the pedal to clip in, and twist your heel out sideways to unclip. They take a little getting used to, but they seriously make you a lot more efficient when you ride. The idea is that you have a stiff shoe sole that's attached to the pedal, so that much more of the energy your legs generate gets used in making the pedals turn and the wheels go round and round.

But I'm getting ahead of myself. Strictly speaking, pedals and cycling shoes are not part of the bare essentials. If you don't feel comfortable with the idea, or don't want to shell out the extra money, you don't have to. Again, my own philosophy is that I'm handicapped in this sport by extra body weight, so I'm going to use the technology to help increase the power that I transfer from my foot to the bike. But it's a personal decision.

Helmet

You gotta have one of these. For one thing, no triathlon will let you out on the course without one. For another, not encasing your brain in an additional protective covering when you're out on any open-topped wheeled conveyance is *stupid. Stupid, stupid, stupid!* My brother-in-law works with lots of folks who weren't wearing helmets when they crashed their motorcycles, bikes, or skateboards. He teaches them to swallow their food again. Maybe learn to talk. So never, never, never go out on your bicycle without a helmet. Have I made myself clear?

Now that we've covered that, the rest is pretty simple. You can get an entry-level helmet for under forty dollars. It should fit snugly, right on top of your head, not slouching down over your eyes or tipped back on your head in a fetching early Audrey Hepburn sort of way. I was watching some kids ride bikes the other day with their helmets (mandatory in California) so far back on their heads that their chin straps appeared to be choking them. I've also seen both kids and adults riding around with their chin straps unfastened. Presumably they think that static electricity will cause the helmet to adhere to their heads during a wipeout. Don't do this. Let the nice young man at the bike store adjust your new brain bucket for you. And then wear it. Always.

Pump

I suppose you could conceivably live without one, but really, this is essential. Actually, you should probably get two pumps, a floor pump for your garage, balcony, sidewalk, or other pre-ride surface, and a frame pump for your bike. The frame pump (or a higher tech equivalent which I'll go into later) should always be attached to your bike when you go out. The floor pump pumps more air so you can easily top up your air pressure and change flats. Doing that stuff regularly with a little skinny frame pump gets old fast. But you can do it. Make sure you buy a pump that fits your tire valves. Presta valves are the skinny little ones with the little doohickey on the end. Schrader valves are exactly the same as your car tire valves. Many pumps have adapters that fit both (for your road bike and your mountain bike, for example). Make sure the nice young woman at the bike store helps you set the pump for the right kind of valve to start out with.

Puncture Repair

It's all very well having a frame pump on your bike, but if you get a flat out on the road (and you *will*), you have to have a few more items to fix it. I carry at least one spare inner tube, preferably two, on any ride because I just loathe the fiddly little process of patching tubes up. Some people are into this. These are usually the people who enjoy "crafting," or building ships in bottles, or other persnickety detail-oriented stuff. Me, I want to slap on a new tube and go. Plus I'm never that confident that my patch is going to hold. But I always have a patch kit in my bike bag just in case. Patch kits are cheap and small.

Then you need something with which to get the tire off your rim and back on again. Again, tire irons are small and cheap. They are also frustrating as hell to use if you happen to have really tight tires on your bike like I do. There are very few alternatives, but I will go into one in the section on Inessential items.

THE RUN: BARE ESSENTIALS

1. Shoes
2. Sports Bra (for women, mostly)

Shoes

Please do not skimp on shoes. You need good shoes that are right for your feet, body type, running style, and goals. To get the right shoes for you, go to a real running store, so you're not trying to get advice on protecting your precious legs and feet from the underpaid kids at the local MegaSport or Big Big Sports Store. Their intentions are good, but they usually don't know the ins and outs of shoe construction or gait and foot analysis like the folks at a real running store. A real running store should have people who know about running, and feet, and strides, and injuries, and how to find you a shoe. They should look at your feet and your stride as you walk and run, and recommend a shoe that keeps your foot in an optimal position for running, provides enough cushioning, and addresses other idiosyncrasies of your feet.

If you identify strongly with the title *Slow Fat Triathlete*, then the right shoe is even more important because your extra poundage is causing extra stress on your feet, and from there on up to your knees, hips, back, and probably to your brain, for all I know. I used to have a lot of little nagging foot injuries until I stopped trying to save money at

MegaBigSport. Once I actually went to the running store and got the shoe they recommended, the foot injuries pretty much went away.

Sports Bra

I look at a good sports bra as an absolute essential for women triathletes. I'm particularly focused on this area since when I started out on the rocky road to fitness back in 1999, I wore a size 46-DDD bra. If I didn't get a very seriously engineered sports bra, I wasn't going to be able to see the road 'cause my breasts would be floppin' up into my face. You may not have this issue, especially if you're male. But if you're a larger-breasted gal, finding the bra with the right amount of support and comfort can make the difference between powering through your workouts and heading for the donut shop in floppy-busted despair. When I'm strapped up tight and ready to go, I feel a lot less self-conscious about going out for my run. The other day, I had to go for a run wearing an old, too-big bra because my industrial-strength bras were too skanky to go out in public. I did about ten minutes and slunk back to the house. I just couldn't deal with the bouncing.

I swear by the Enell sports bra—it's not the most stylish thing out there, but boy does it hold you in place. One catalog refers to it as the "bra of last resort." I always catch myself humming "Ride of the Valkyries" as I wrestle my way into one. It's got wide shoulder straps, it hooks up the front, and it lasts forever. Champion, Nike, Hind, and Moving Comfort also make good stuff. So go get something good.

INESSENTIAL, BUT NICE TO HAVE

THE SWIM: INESSENTIALS

OK, you have your suit, your goggles, and maybe even a wetsuit. What else might you want to round out your gear bag for swimming? Not much. This is really the most stripped down of the three disciplines, literally and figuratively.

Swim Cap

You'll probably get a latex swim cap at your very first race. Most races give you color-coded caps so you know which group you're starting with. The latex caps are fine for racing or emergency use, but they are kind of cheap and flimsy, with a feel like a deflated party balloon. I use a silicone cap when I'm training. It keeps the hair out of my face and I like to think it protects my glamorous tresses from getting fried by chlorine. Silicone doesn't seem to grab at my hair the way that the latex does; it has a smoother, more pliable feel, and it's also a lot more durable. Clearly, however, we are looking at fine points here. The swim cap also contributes to the AquaTriWoman/FrogTriMan effect.

Earplugs

A lot of people have problems with water getting in their ears when they swim a bunch. I myself spend large chunks of time with my hearing somewhat impaired by water sloshing around in there. Sometimes if the water's cold, it can really make your ears hurt. Earlier this spring, at my first race of the season, I bought some silicone earplugs to wear in the frigid water. It worked to keep my ears comfy, but I had a hard time removing them with my frozen fingers, so that was a mixed success. There are also "flange" earplugs that make you look like you're growing caterpillars in your ears. Go ahead and experiment.

THE BIKE: INESSENTIALS

Bike Shorts

I don't get on a bike without some extra padding between the saddle and my posterior. But that's just me. I'm a Leo and I like my butt to be comfortable. You can easily train enough for a sprint-distance tri without padded bike shorts. If you end up wanting to go on longer rides and do longer races, bike shorts become pretty essential. Some people are embarrassed to go outside in form-fitting Lycra shorts. You can buy padded undershorts that you can wear underneath something baggy if you want. But the longer you ride, the less you want baggy stuff flapping around, bunching up and chafing, and providing greater wind resistance. (You may choose to go straight for a pair of tri shorts, which have thinner, lighter padding so, come race day, you can wear them for swim, bike, and run and not feel like you're wearing a diaper. See the section on tri clothing under General Inessentials.)

Gloves

Again, I have to have my padded gloves for even a short ride. Some people ride the bike leg of Olympic distance and longer triathlons without them. The padding protects your hands from pressure and vibration, plus the gloves give you interesting tan lines. There are fingerless gloves for warmer weather, and, for you denizens of the Arctic, they make full-on fleecy, windproofed, fingerfull gloves with nice little grippy bits on the fingertips so you can still control your brakes and shifters.

Bike Computer

I have a hard time categorizing this as inessential but I know I'm a little bit of a geek. I find it's just so fascinating to know how far I've ridden, what my average speed is, whether my current speed is faster or slower than the average, what my high speed is, how many miles I've ridden since I first started riding this bike. . . . Like I said, a little geeky. But a lot of folks who get into triathlon do like their little measuring devices. You may not want one.

Cycling Shoes and Clipless Pedals

I talked a little bit about these in the bike essentials section. Lots of people do their first races by riding in their running shoes. It certainly saves you time on transitions when you don't have to change shoes after the bike leg. Many people are nervous about being cleated into a pedal. They feel like they won't be able to get their feet out fast enough when they need to put a foot on the ground and then they'll topple over like a statue of Lenin in 1991.

A cycling shoe/clipless pedal combo offers a lot of advantages though, just like wetsuits.

1. You transfer more force to the pedals. Cycling shoes have stiff soles, which give you more leverage on the pedal. Say you wanted to move a one-hundred-pound boulder with a lever. Would you pick a flexible rubber lever? I don't think so. Well, your running shoes are a flexible rubber lever for applying force to the pedals. You waste a lot of energy with that.

2. You can develop a more efficient pedaling stroke. When you have cycling shoes that are attached to your clipless pedals with an easy-to-use cleat system, you can start to learn to pedal in circles. You might think that the pedals already go in circles. That's exactly right. But people don't naturally follow that circular motion with their feet and legs. They stomp down on the pedal on one side, then stomp down on the other side. If they try anything else, their shoes come off the pedals, and suddenly there's no pedaling at all. But when your shoes and your feet and your pedals are firmly

attached to each other, your feet can follow the pedals, and you can apply pressure throughout most of their motion.

3. You can walk around making clippety-clop noises with your cleats when you stop for coffee after the ride. This impresses the heck out of people. Or at least you can think that.

4. You will develop a heretofore-unimaginable level of foot coordination learning to get your feet in and out of your pedals without falling over. And, as with the wetsuit above, your contortions will amuse onlookers. No, seriously, don't worry about this part of it. A few minutes of practice and you'll be able to handle it well enough. Getting the feet out is easy. I'm a complete klutz and I still figured out how to do it without falling over once. I still scramble to get clipped in occasionally, but I'm sure another few years of riding will take care of that.

Bike Jersey

I resisted this for a long time. "I don't need no fancy graphics and back pockets," I insisted. I rode for a long time in a T-shirt, albeit a high-tech wicking fabric T-shirt, or a tank top. But then my tri club offered club jerseys for sale, and I succumbed to the urge to identify with the pack. First of all, the profusion of club sponsor logos and the bright colors instantly made me feel faster and more serious. The fabric was sleek and silky, and the three big pockets across the back were incredibly useful. I could slam keys, ID, energy bars, and even my cell phone in there. Hell, I could carry peanut butter and jelly sandwiches! If your training rides never go over an hour, you can easily get by without spending the money on a bike jersey. For longer stuff, yeah, it makes life easier and more comfortable.

Water Bottles and Cages

Hydration is your friend. The only reason that I'm not including this with bare essentials is that you could conceivably manage without if you never ride your bike for more than an hour, and you make sure you drink copiously before and after your ride. Or stick a water bottle down your shorts. Or stop for bottled water every forty-five minutes or so. But why make it complicated? Water bottles, and the cages that hold them onto your bike, are cheap and easy to manage. Go ahead and get some. Get big water bottles with wide mouths so you can throw ice cubes or powdered drink mixes in them. Or you could get a Camelbak or similar "hydration backpack." These are backpacks which hold a big ol' bladder for the water or other liquid and a tube so you can drink while you ride, not even taking your hand from the handlebars. We'll talk more later about hydrating when you exercise. For now, just trust me.

Allen Wrenches

Most of the stuff on your bike that gets loose needs either a three-, four-, or five-millimeter allen or hex wrench to tighten up. The bike stores and catalogs sell other multitasking bike tools that you can take with you on your ride, but you might feel pressure to learn what the other tools are for. Spoke wrench? Chain tool? One of these days I should probably learn what those are for and how to use them. But for now I ride around with a hardware store set of allen wrenches.

Bike Bag

You've spent all this other money, now go out and get a little bag that fits under your seat and holds your spare tube(s), patch kit, tire irons, a couple of gels, a couple bucks of snack money, and your allen wrench.

THE RUN: INESSENTIALS

Frivolous socks

Seriously, these are one of my favorite parts of triathlon. You don't have to be a triathlete to wear them, or even wear them to be a triathlete, but the cycling/running socks adorned with chili peppers, chameleons, happy faces, skulls and crossbones, or the biohazard symbol seem to be pretty common at rides, races, and track workouts. They're just plain fun. If you feel that silly socks are demeaning to your dignity, you can get plain old white or black ones. Party pooper. Just keep in mind that triathlon is designed to strip you of that kind of appearance-related faux dignity, as your first encounter with a wetsuit will prove.

Here's a piece of advice I'm passing on from a foot doctor, podiatrist, whatever you call 'em: Get thin socks. It's really easy, when you see the thick, cushy socks with the extra thick loops on the bottom, to think, "Yeah, that's what I need, extra padding." I bought these socks for years, thinking I was doing my feet a favor. Then I figured out that if I needed extra padding in my socks so my feet didn't hurt, I should probably just get better shoes. Once I switched to thin socks, my toes suddenly felt much less cramped and crowded in the running shoes.

Oh, and let me just state the obvious: Don't run in cotton socks. In fact, don't do anything in cotton socks that makes your feet sweat. Soggy, wet, blistered, unhappy feet, nasty, ick. Of course, if you already do run ten miles a day in your cotton gym socks, carry on, don't mind me. But I firmly believe God created synthetic fabrics for endurance athletes and wanna be endurance athletes. It's the least we can do to use them. DeFeet, The Sock Guy, Lin, SmartWool, Ironman, and many other brands offer excellent socks, both frivolous and stolid.

Fancy Wicking Clothing

Prepare yourself for another anti-cotton diatribe. Working out in cotton basically sucks. It gets wet when you sweat, it gets heavy, it gets cold if you get cold, and it bunches up and chafes. Like all zealots, I am a convert from the other side. I used to run in cotton T-shirts. In fact, when my friend Russ bought his first CoolMax shirt, I called him a "f*&#ing gearhead." I need to learn to quit making fun of people, because I always turn into those exact same people as time goes by. I used to make fun of people with cell phones, too. Now I have both a cell phone and a drawer full of fancy wicking fabrics. Anyhow, the nifty synthetic fabrics that are used now to make running shorts, shirts, and tri-wear are just too darn comfortable and practical to pass up. They keep you warmer when you need to be warm, drier, and cooler when you need to be cool. They're featherlight and they glide over your body in a lovely sensuous way. I'm hooked.

Elastic Laces or Lace Locks

I like to tell my running friends that triathletes are people who can't tie their shoes. But thanks to technology we don't have to. A few companies make these nifty devices that let you get your running shoes on and off in a hurry. Obviously you don't need these for your first triathlon, but I love them so much I'm tempted to put them on all my shoes. Elastic laces! Amazing! I like Yankz, others swear by SpeedLaces, each of which has a neat little clip system. There are also laces just like regular shoelaces, except elastic. And there are these plastic clip gizmos that go on to your regular laces so you don't have to tie a knot. I think elastic's better. It's faster to get on and it adjusts to your foot better while you're running. These inexpensive gadgets make your bike-to-run transition a heck of a lot easier. In fact, for me they even make it easier to go out for a training run. Just knowing I can pull my shoes on without tying two knots is one less mental barrier to overcome when I come home from the office all tired and grumpy and I still need to get a run in.

GENERAL INESSENTIALS

Sunglasses

Particularly important on the bike, where wind, bugs, dust, and road debris can really irritate or endanger the windows of the soul. Get the wraparound kind for more protection. If you're like me, buy multiple cheap pairs. I lose sunglasses like senior citizens lose money in Vegas.

Sport watch

It's nice to be able to keep track of how slowly you're going. Especially as you begin to improve and find yourself going less slowly. I started out timing my runs wearing my dressy little chain-link watch, but it was hard to see that tiny dial and also see where I was going in the field by the park. So for thirty-five bucks or so, I got a sleek Timex unit that counts laps, has a stopwatch function, and does a couple other things I haven't bothered to figure out yet. It's fine in the water, it has the cool Indiglo night-light; it's great. I'm not the sports watch connoisseur that Russ is. Maybe I'll go interview him for his views on sports watches for the next edition of this book.

Tri Shorts and Other Race Wear

This gear comes under the heading of inessentials because lots of people race without them. But I would recommend tri shorts even for your first race. They're basically bike shorts with a little less padding than regular bike shorts, made out of one of the many wonderful varieties of quick-dry material. If you want to be really efficient with your gear purchasing, you can use tri shorts for all your bike rides. You can get them for somewhere around thirty or forty dollars from a number of locations and online emporia, which I'll list in the Appendix. You can pair them with a specialized triathlon top, a bike jersey, a synthetic workout top, a sports bra, or, if you really insist, a cotton T-shirt. But you know how I feel about cotton for working out.

For my first race, I wore tri shorts and a CoolMax tank top under my wetsuit. I was very comfortable and I didn't have to worry about adding or subtracting any clothing once the wetsuit was off. Then I started racing in my bike jersey 'cause I wanted to fly my club colors. This was pretty good except the sleeves chafed when I ran. You may have already noticed that chafing features prominently in my narrative. It's bad enough for skinny triathletes, but when you add extra flesh into the equation, eliminating chafing becomes an obsession. Eventually I got a sleeveless triathlon top with a cute little pocket in the back, and that was a good thing. It was a men's top, of course—I still don't fit into any women's sizes of tri tops—but you know, who's checking up on this? The triathlon apparel police? Hell no!

Energy Gels and Bars

Clif Bars, PowerBars, Luna Bars, Pria Bars, Odwalla Bars, Harvest Bars—there are more energy bars out there than you can shake a stick at. And there are handy little foil packets of carbohydrate-rich gel, usually about a hundred calories a serving, that you can suck down as you're running or cycling. If you're working out for under an hour, don't even worry about gels. They are pretty convenient, though, for long workouts and races. And energy bars are always somewhere around my person—in my purse, in my gym bag, in my desk drawer, melting in my car, whatever.

Sports Drinks

Water's good, definitely. For workouts that are less than an hour long, which for your first sprint-distance tri should be most all of them, water's probably all you need to stay hydrated and happy. When you sweat, though, you do lose things that you need to replace. Sodium, potassium, magnesium, manganese, the whole darn chemistry lesson, otherwise known as electrolytes. Your body needs them to be in balance, otherwise things can get seriously out of whack. Like your heart can quit beating in its accustomed rhythm.

You can replace electrolytes after short workouts by eating a varied, balanced diet that includes things like fruits, veggies, low-fat dairy, fish, tofu, lean meats, whole grains. Or you can eat Twinkies and multivitamins, but I don't think you'll feel quite as good. More on this later. Should you feel the need to get some calories and electrolytes into you in liquid form, there are all kinds of sports drinks on the market, from Gatorade to G-Push to Hammer Nutrition's Perpetuum, formulated with Chromium Polynicotinate, Tribasic Sodium Phosphate, and Carnosine, a naturally occurring dipeptide from the amino acids histidine and alanine. Huh?

For the novice triathlete, Hammer Nutrition might be overkill. The word on the street is that Hammer's products are the bomb for long distance training and racing, but you probably just don't need that much science when you're starting out. Myself, I drink quite a bit of Cytomax (another brand) for workouts that are longer than about ninety minutes, and yet another brand's product called Endurox R4 after long hard workouts or races. The Cytomax hydrates great and gives me energy, and the Endurox really does seem to help me recover faster after a strenuous effort. By this I mean that my muscles are less sore the next day and I don't have that drained, tapped-out feeling.

You can talk to twenty different triathletes and get twenty-five different opinions on sports drinks. Gatorade works fine, too. If you want to get into the fancier formulas, get smaller sizes or samples if you can. Use it during and after your workouts and see if it agrees with you or if it makes your stomach cramp or heave. See if it gives you a nice energy boost or a big old sugar rush followed by the shakes.

BodyGlide

This water-based lubricant is not the best for bedroom encounters (see AstroLube and some other book for that), but it works really well to help you get your wetsuit on and off and to avoid chafing at the neck of the wetsuit. You can apply it anywhere on your body where you might experience chafing during the swim, bike, or run. Use your imagination. After you've trained for a few weeks, you won't need your imagination—you'll know all your hot spots for the chafe. Bodyglide comes in original formula or with sunscreen. Only buy the sunscreen Bodyglide if you want to experience an odor approximating rancid whale blubber. Ick. There are lots of other lube-y solutions out there that you can try, too, if Bodyglide doesn't meet your individual needs. Just make sure anything you wear under your wetsuit is safe for the rubber. Petroleum-based products like Vaseline can make the Neoprene deteriorate. If in doubt, don't use it.

FUN STUFF FOR SWIMMING, CYCLING, RUNNING, AND RACING

Aerobars

These are the additions to regular handlebars that stick out in front like little horns. You rest your elbows down on the elbow pads, stick your hands out forward, and whoosh! You look just like Jan Ullrich riding a time trial. Aerobars allow you to get down in a low, sleek, aerodynamic position, thereby expending less energy to go faster. Only on a road bike though. If you have a mountain bike or a beach cruiser, the Official Code of Cycling Accessories mandates that you not put aerobars on it because there's very little that's aerodynamic about your bike anyway. However, as I am all in favor of general dorkiness, and triathlon dorkiness in particular, go ahead and do it if you get the urge.

Bento Box

These are really cute little nylon and webbing contraptions that strap onto the top tube of your bike (that's the one parallel to the ground, for those keeping score) and hold gel packets, energy bars, whatever you might wish to snack on during your long ride or race. I love that they're called "Bento," after the neat boxes that divide up Japanese meals into sushi, tempura, cutlets, and so on. Despite my enthusiasm for the product, I have not yet succumbed to the temptation to get one. If you ride a "girl's bike" with two slanty tubes, this isn't going to work so well for you either.

Telescoping Tire Tool

An awesome stocking stuffer. Works even better than traditional tire irons, which is to say, hardly at all if your tire is tight on your rim. For a complete explanation of how to change a tire, I'm going to let some other poor sucker take the responsibility. But in my experience, the telescoping tire tool and a lot of PAM spray or spit can help slide a recalcitrant tire over the rim. Lubrication and leverage beat brute force most every time.

CO$_2$ System

This is a great toy for those among us who like to blow up balloons till they pop and make the cat run for cover. You know who you are. You know those little CO$_2$ cartridges that you can buy in the hardware store or the paintball supply shop? Well, you can buy an adaptor for those that will fit onto your tire valve and inflate your tire in seconds. I never want to use a frame pump again now that I have the CO$_2$ gun. Especially since I've had some sad experiences with frame pumps, which I will describe in excruciating detail in the race report at the end of this chapter. The one drawback to them is that once you're out of cartridges in your bike bag, you're done; whereas with a properly fitted frame pump and a bunch of elbow grease, you can pump up as many punctures as you can patch.

Neoprene Seat Cover

For the tender of tushie, the Neoprene seat cover is a delightful invention. It slides on over your saddle like a thick stretchy condom (and should be applied in the same inside-out rolling manner) and protects your nether regions from vibration and other wear and tear. If you wear padded bike shorts, you may or may not want to experiment with these. I find them helpful in races because my tri shorts have lighter padding than my regular bike shorts.

Race Belt

I love my race belt because I'm really hopeless with safety pins. In my opinion, the very name "safety pin" is thoroughly misleading. I have always been prone to inflicting painful puncture wounds in my fingers, thumbs, and even torso when attempting to "safety" pin my race numbers to my race clothes. And why put holes in your fancy tri gear anyway? The race belt is a simple band of elastic webbing with a buckle on it and a couple of fasteners that hold your race number. You can put it on under your wetsuit, or you can grab it in transition as you head out onto the bike or run. I usually wait until the run because the number flaps around a lot on the bike. Another advantage of this device is that you can rotate your number to the back for most of the race, where flapping won't bother you, and then bring it round to the front at the end, where the race announcers and photographers are.

Seal Mask

I haven't succumbed to the lure of this toy yet, but I probably will some day. It's basically swim goggles on steroids. Larger lenses give you a better, less distorted view of your watery surroundings. This can be useful when navigation is an issue, like when you can't see the buoys on the course because of sun, fog, or rain.

OK, I could probably go on and on about equipment, but instead I'll close with a cautionary tale about puncture repair in a race situation.

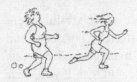

Pump It Up!

May 19, 2002
Uvas South Bay Triathlon: 1,200-yard swim | 16-mile bike | 5-mile run
Uvas Reservoir, Morgan Hill, California

Fifteen days after an ecstatic triathlon debut at Wildflower, your intrepid correspondent sets off down highway Eighty-Five, a few minutes behind schedule at 6:08 A.M. The Uvas tri is a smaller, more local event, seven hundred participants in all, tucked away among the hills south of San Jose.

It's a big step for me. The twelve-hundred-yard swim is three times my Wildflower splash. The sixteen-mile bike ride is pretty easy (except for Sycamore Hill, which kicked my booty on my practice ride), but the five-mile run seems awfully long for someone with a nagging lower back issue.

This is my second tri, so I'm more casual in my race-day approach. But the drive's longer than I remembered and hordes of people are waiting to turn into the lot, so by the time I hit my rack, it's only an hour before start time, and I have so much socializing to accomplish! Our mighty Silicon Valley Triathlon Club makes up 10 percent of the total entries in the race so there are *many* people to greet and encourage. Plus best-tri-buddy Russ, of course.

Fifteen minutes before my wave start, I'm having funky logistics. The greased-pig wetsuit routine goes OK, but I forget to take my rings off and have to run back. I misplace my goggles and find them on the back of a support cart. Volunteers are bellowing, "All racers clear the transition area!" But I'm not *ready* yet! OK, OK, I'm done. I'm at the start.

The Uvas Reservoir and surroundings are gorgeous. We have to swim around a cute bulbous peninsula—easy as pie to stay on course, right? Um, yeah. Oh, I was supposed to go around *that* orange buoy? That one back there? Thanks . . . So that adds about seventy-five yards to my swim. Boy, twelve hundred plus seventy-five yards at 8 A.M. seems really long. I have no idea where I am in the pack, but I fear the worst. Finally I dare to look behind me. There are people there! From my wave! Wow. Encouraged, I turn it on a little and smile for the cameras as I emerge from the water. Ouch! Ouch! Ouch! That battered parking lot has way too much topography for my feet.

The wetsuit seems stubborn coming off, or my arms are tired. It's a cloudy day, not too warm, so my sodden tri shorts and bike jersey provide more evaporative cooling than I would like. Heading onto the road I spot my mom cheering me on. The bike course is lovely, and I'm averaging 16.5 miles per hour, faster than I hoped. Are my spiffy new Michelin Kevlar-lined, high-pressure tires the cause? Must be. Great tires. Yay. This is a great race!

Halfway through the bike course I misjudge a ninety-degree turn and only stay upright by going off road for a few yards. Pride in my nifty bike handling turns to chagrin as I realize that the vibration under my rear is not rough asphalt. A flat in my spiffy new Kevlar-lined tires? Never fear! I pop my spare tube in and even get the tire back on the rim without much trouble. But my pump won't fit on the valve! Ack! Have I never used this pump before? Surely I wouldn't have gone on a race with a pump I haven't used . . . Dang.

A transcendent, highly evolved, kind woman stops and loans me her pump. I can see instantly it will fit my valve. (Thanks, Number 20.) But I can't figure out how to lock it on. Struggle, fruitless pumping, lots of cursing, and the hissing of escaping air. Finally I get it—the lock lever goes the *other way*. Now I'm good. I cram all the air I can into the offending tube, unlock the pump, and pull it off. To my horror, the pump takes my valve head with it. All the precious compressed air is back in the atmosphere, and the valve head is rattling around inside the pump, rendering it useless. I'm hosed. And I've broken this goddess's pump. And all the other bikes have passed me by.

Do I want to push my bike for another eight miles so I can have the chance of finishing this race in, oh, five hours or so? Mmmmm . . . no. Besides, I fear the effect on my parents' nerves if I fail to show up at the transition. So I flag down yet another beautiful, transcendent goddess, this one in a pickup, and hitch a ride back to near the transition. (Thanks, Katherine.) By this time I'm so bummed and brain-locked that I can't figure out how to get my rear wheel back on, so I start carrying my bike back to base. This walk must be at least four miles. Mentally, anyway.

Dejected, I turn the last bend and see Russ, my mom and dad, and Chris from SVTC, all hustling toward me. Relieved that I am unbloodied and unbroken, they give out hugs, help me put my bike away, and offer consoling words like, "You mean you didn't *know* if your pump worked with your tires??" Chris pats me on the back and says, "Come on, you've got a run to do!"

The little joyride in the pickup disqualified me from an official finish, but I still need to do that five-mile run. For one thing, I've planned on a good hard workout today, and I'll feel even more disappointed if I go home less than completely exhausted. Plus I'm feeling like crap and I need to get some endorphins going. And I feel stubborn about it. But the thought of an hour out on the course as the last runner to set out isn't too appealing.

Still, I trot out the gate and down the little hill, keeping my feet moving, trying to keep an OK pace. To my astonishment, I catch a sixty-six-year-old woman at mile two, and two more women at the turnaround. But that's all. Everyone else is ahead of me. Departing finishers wave and honk to cheer me on. I feel embarrassed. I've DNF'ed (did not finish); I'm not really the gallant slowpoke they think I am. I had a forty-five-minute break and didn't ride Sycamore Hill. (And if I had ridden the rest of the course, I'd have finished long ago, thank you very much.) But maybe I'm gallant in my own foolish way. I worked my butt off to get as far as I did. I struggled mightily with my mechanical and mental failures, and I'm still goin'.

The endorphins work magic. My crushed spirit regains its shape and I even muster another smile at the finish line. I'll call it my Uvas Du-and-a-half-athlon. I savor the bananas and juices of moral victory at the post-race bash and plod off to the car with Mom and Dad—the best race support crew ever. In a perfect parental moment, a moist towelette appears out of Mom's purse to help me get the worst of the bike grease off.

I head north on eighty-five, still liberally marked with bike grease and redolent of lake water. A sadder but wiser du-and-a-half-athlete, I am just as exhausted as I wanted to be, and it still seems like it was a pretty darn good morning.

Next on the odyssey—Tri For Fun in Pleasanton, June 15. Back to the sprint distance. Still have to figure out how my frame pump works. Can't wait!

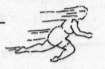

The Slow Fat Triathlete
Recommends

Well, pretty much this whole chapter is recommendations of one sort or another. The few key points for me are:

1. Start Minimalist. Buy the very least amount of gear that you need to do your first race in reasonable comfort. You can always buy more. And if you get into triathlon like I did, you will buy more. Much more. But I'm still riding the $378 bike I bought off eBay because it works just fine. And because I've only been able to find part-time work for over a year now thanks to the continuing icky economy here in Silicon Valley.
2. Have Fun With Your Small Purchases. If it makes you feel good to have a pair of bright turquoise tri shorts and coordinating Iron Girl socks, by all means go for it. You may need to do fun stuff to balance out the discipline and rigors of training.

3. Take Advice with a Grain of Salt. Definitely seek out input from other triathletes or folks at the bike store or running shoe store, but don't take it as gospel. You don't *need* anything except a bike that works, a helmet, and some shoes you can run in. Oh, and something to swim in. That's it. The rest is just making yourself comfortable, a little faster, and/or a little more stylish. You decide how much you need to spend to accomplish those goals.

4. Having Said That: Don't downplay your need to be comfortable when you train and race. With things like shoes and bike fit, comfort is a necessity—if you're not comfortable, you will probably get injured and jeopardize your nascent triathlon career. If your socks make your feet feel squished or give you blisters, it's another demotivator. So is having your cotton gym shorts chafe between your thighs. In my world, the more comfortable I am when I'm training, the more likely I am to enjoy it, and the more likely I am to keep doing it. And the more out of shape you are, the more likely you are to have to pay special attention to issues like chafing and having your bike fit you just right. When you're twenty years old and lean as a greyhound, you can handle less-than-adequate shoes for a while. When you're forty and tubby like me, it just ain't gonna work.

5. Try Stuff On. Don't worry about being thought demanding or diva-esque. Try everything on, try it in multiple sizes and styles—make that sales associate work for his puny wage. This gear has to work for you, so make sure it fits and functions just right.

4
TRAINING DAZE

PREPARING YOURSELF
TO ACTUALLY DO THIS

ALL RIGHT, YOU'VE made the commitment to doing a triathlon, and you've figured out how much of your precious bank account you're going to blow on the gear, at least at first. (Or else you're one of those armchair triathletes who have no intention of ever doing a race. You just like reading about other people's suffering. It's OK, as long as you bought this book, I'm happy.) Now all you have to do is get your body and mind trained to do the race. Believe it or not, the training is kind of the easy part, once you've made your mind up you're going to do it. You just have to figure out a schedule that lets you swim, bike, and run every week, preferably fitting in each sport at least twice. Simple, huh?

OK, I'm lying again. It's not *that* easy to create and maintain a training plan. It's not even that easy to do random workouts most days of the week. And if you're a typically overscheduled American with a full-time job, a passel of young 'uns with soccer, ballet, tutoring, and swim team practices, and a house to take care of, the idea of signing up for activities that consume even more hours in the week is pretty daunting. But you can do it. I don't know how, since I currently have neither a full-time job, kids, nor a house, but I know it can be done 'cause lots of people in my tri club have all of the above, and they still kick my butt at both training and racing.

Kelly told me she mostly just runs, and squeezes swimming and biking in when she can. Ahmet, who competes at a high level locally, does one workout in the morning before work and another one at lunchtime. Dave says that once you make the commitment to being active, you'll figure out how to fit it in. The important thing is to "treat yourself *first* to physical activity—all of your dependents and partners will benefit by your increased happiness." Some moms and dads jog around the perimeter of the soccer field while their kids practice, or if they have young children, they plunk them in the sand pit of the long jump while they run around the track.

And of course there's my personal triathlon hero, Gina Kehr. She combines the rigorous training regimen of a top pro with a full-time job as a real-estate agent. And she still finds time to work as assistant track coach for the Silicon Valley Tri Club. Clearly she has the energy of a hummingbird and the drive of a Hummer, but it's something for us mortals to emulate.

Again, the reason that I can't use my own example to inspire you here is that I have a totally sweet setup. I work three-quarter time, with flexible hours, for a very cool employer about ten minutes from my house. My husband supports my triathlon obsession with benign serenity, and he loves to cook dinner, too. He has a superhuman tolerance for my natural slobbiness and tendency to strew sweaty workout clothes and bottles of stagnant water around the house and patio area. I also live in the Bay Area of California, in an area with an almost perfect year-round climate and an abundance of great places to train. So I have it made, I admit.

For me, the biggest obstacle to training is morning. I don't face it well, never have. Not only am I congenitally averse to getting up in the morning, I can't really stay up late either. Left to my own devices, I sleep a solid nine and a half hours a night, and a demanding training plan just makes me even more determined to get my Zs in. Any training plan that calls for pre-dawn workouts is dead in the water as far as I'm concerned. I decided to test my limits last summer and signed up for four Tuesday morning swim clinics that started at 6 A.M. I made it to three of them, which was a triumph, but I had to come home from work at noon and nap for two hours each time. So if I advise you to fit your workouts in by "just getting up a little earlier in the morning," please note that I am speaking in purest "do as I say, not as I do" mode, and feel free to sneer at my hypocrisy. It is an option though, if you like that morning sort of thing. The only inspiration I hope my story can offer is that you can be both butt-lazy and still train your ass enough to get through some triathlons. It works for me.

WEATHER

EVEN HERE IN the mild climate of Northern California, I hear some people bitching about the weather. "Oh, it's too hot to run," or "I just hate swimming when it's raining." Babies. And I'm pretty sure that there's a lot more reason to bitch about the weather if you live in Buffalo, or Sioux Falls, or in Florida in August. Obviously you have to take local conditions into account when you set up your training program. Maybe figure out where you can swim when it's forty below out there. Get yourself some nice thick polypro tights so you can run when it's cold, snowing, sleeting, whatever it does where you are. When it's hot and humid, try not to do your hardest workouts during the full blazing heat of the day. You have common sense; you manage your meteorological challenges in your everyday life. My request to you is that you look at getting outside your regular comfort zone a little when it comes to exercise and the climate. So maybe it's raining? I love swimming in the rain. Hey, I'm gonna get wet anyway. See if you can have an adventure with the weather and your workout. Cold and wet is temporary, as long as you get warm and dry when you get home. Have some fun with it.

SCHEDULING

WHAT WITH WORK and the weather and all, you need to figure some things out about when and where you're going to get your workouts in. And you need to schedule in some time off. When you're starting out, it's particularly important to give your body and mind some rest days—at least one a week.

One rule of thumb that has worked for me is to spend more time on my weaknesses. For most of my triathlon career so far, running has been my weakest link. So I try and get three runs in every week. Cycling is my strongest sport, so if I have to skip a workout, it's probably going to be a bike ride. Swimming used to be my middle sport, but since I've worked hard on my running, swimming has now become my worst. So this off-season I'm planning to spend more time in the pool.

If you're just starting in all three sports, or you feel equally competent or incompetent in all of them, shoot for two workouts in each during the course of the week. Maybe block out something like this to start off with for your first four weeks:

Week One

TOTAL HOURS: 2:45

Monday	Tuesday	Wednesday	Thursday	Friday	Saturday	Sunday
Off	Run :20	Swim :30	Bike :40	Run :25	Swim :30	Bike :45

Week Two

TOTAL HOURS: 3:00

Monday	Tuesday	Wednesday	Thursday	Friday	Saturday	Sunday
Off	Run :25	Swim :30	Bike :40	Run :30	Swim :30	Bike :50

Week Three

TOTAL HOURS: 3:45

Monday	Tuesday	Wednesday	Thursday	Friday	Saturday	Sunday
Off	Run :30	Swim :30	Bike :45	Run :30	Swim :30	Bike :60

Week Four

TOTAL HOURS: 3:20

Monday	Tuesday	Wednesday	Thursday	Friday	Saturday	Sunday
Off	Run :20	Swim :30	Bike :45	Run: 30	Swim :30	Bike: 45

You don't have to do the same things on the same days every week, either. You could take your day off in the middle of the week, or on Friday, or whenever. The main thing that I would advise here is to rotate your workouts rather than doing run-run, swim-swim, bike-bike. Alternating sports gives your various muscle groups, joints, and ligaments a chance to rest and get stronger before you hit them again. You'll also see that I would have you increase the time you work out very gradually, especially in running, and that the fourth week is actually a step back in workload to allow your body to consolidate the fitness gains of the first three weeks. Both of these are really good rules to follow for as long as you train. Most running coaches say that you shouldn't increase your running workload by more than 10 percent a week, and that you should back off your mileage every few weeks.

The intensity of your running, also, should be very low, very mellow, if you're just starting out. Consider carrying a margarita or mai tai with you as you run to remind you of just how easy this should be. Run slowly, with small strides, and try and keep your breathing easy enough so that you can breathe in during the course of three strides, then breathe out for three strides. If you have to breathe harder than that, slow down or walk, then try again.

As far as swimming goes, if you haven't been swimming regularly, work up to to getting to the pool two days a week and swimming for a solid thirty minutes each time. If you do this for four weeks, you should see some pretty good improvement by the end of the fourth week.

Now, every swim coach will say, "Oh, you should be in the pool at least four times a week to develop your feel for the water." Yeah, well, that would be nice, but it's never happened for me. I talked to one woman in my club who swims once a week at most. I get two or three swims in, depending on what my coach tells me to do. Some people love swimming and swim every day, year round. Similarly, the running coach for my club's New to the Sport program runs almost every day. I find that if I run more than four times a week, I start to feel pretty beat up from the pounding of my weight on the pavement. Same with cycling. You don't get the pounding from impact, but you do put strain on your back, neck, and shoulders, as well as using muscles in your hips and legs that can tighten up if you overuse them.

So I guess what I'm trying to say is when you're starting the training process, err on the side of underworking yourself rather than overworking. I think you'll gain more fitness and have more fun if you mix up your workouts and *don't* go too hard in the beginning.

EASY, EASY, EASY

PROBABLY THE NUMBER one thing that I would tell you to do, and I know that pretty much every coach would agree with me, is to increase your exercise workload gradually. Go easy on yourself at first. I've done this to myself more times than I can tell you: I get enthusiastic, I start working out, I do too much, I hurt myself, and I'm back on the couch, frustrated and well on my way to gaining another ten pounds. You need to go easy on your feet, your knees, your back, your hips, your hamstrings, your shoulders, and pretty much everything in between, too.

One of the biggest challenges in triathlon is the discipline of patience.

You can't get there in a day or a week, maybe not even in a year, depending on where your starting point is and what your goals are. I have a goal to do an Ironman distance race (140.6 miles altogether), but it's probably not going to be until my fourth season of training and racing. Your age, your weight, your previous athletic experience, your injury history, your medical conditions—all factor into how patient you're going to have to be. If you're battling high blood pressure, your doctor may advise you to approach exercise with more caution. If you're twenty-five, fit, lean, and springy, and you can jump on your bike and go for two hours, then you can get going in a triathlon with only a couple of months' preparation, maybe less. And bless you for buying my book because you obviously don't need it.

I'm not a personal trainer or exercise physiologist, but I have trained a lot and been injured a lot. In the course of my recovery and rehabbing, I've learned a little bit about getting stronger versus getting hurt and what your body does when you work out. The basic idea is that when you do some exercise, you stress your muscles and the tendons and ligaments that hold your bones and muscles in place. This stress expresses itself in little teeny tears in the fibers of those muscles and ligaments. If you stress yourself just a little bit and then give your body time to rest and recover, your body will respond by repairing the tears, or microtraumas, and making the whole stressed area stronger. If you stress those muscles all at once, you'll risk incurring more and bigger traumas to the muscle that your body won't be able to repair before you go out and stress it again. You could pull a hamstring, tweak your back, or strain a calf muscle. If you keep stressing the same muscles over and over again and don't give yourself a rest, you risk overuse injuries like tendonitis; plantar fascitis, where your heel hurts for a really long time; or a chronically sore back.

The nifty little secret of triathlon is that you can work different muscles and joints in different ways on different days so you can spread out the stress. If you run on Tuesday, swim on Wednesday, bike on Thursday, and don't run again till Friday, you may just fool your knees, feet, and back into thinking they've had two days of rest. Which they have—at least from running.

And when you go out for every workout, start really slowly. Take the first ten minutes or so to warm up gradually, at an easy pace, not straining anything at all. And make sure you cool down for at least ten minutes at the end. The mathematically inclined among you will note that, for a twenty-minute run, that means you just warm up and cool down.

This is correct. At first, when twenty minutes is all you can do, it should pretty much all be at a very easy, comfortable pace.

HOW MUCH TIME DO I NEED TO GET READY?

I HAVE NO idea. You might be in good enough shape to jump off the couch and go do an Olympic distance race. Or you might be a lifelong couch dweller who needs to relearn how to ride a bike. It depends on your age, your body's resiliency, your past history of exercise, your weight, your strength, your endurance, the distance and terrain of the race—in short pretty much everything can affect how much lead time you need to prepare safely for a triathlon. If you're slow, fat, old, and inexperienced, a year might not be too much lead time for you. If you have a history of back problems, for example, or high cholesterol, or you've been diagnosed with diabetes, you need to check with your doc about any of this. The absolutely critical thing is not to rush your preparation. Allow enough time that you build up your fitness in all three sports slowly and safely. When in doubt, go slower, do less, take more time.

TRIATHLETE'S LOG, STARDATE 2004.6.1

NOT TO GET all Trekkie-geeky about it, but I think keeping a training log is a great thing. You will learn a lot about yourself and your body if you write down every workout you do, how long it was, how intense it was, how you felt, and whatever other data seems relevant to you. Your log also gives your training a sense of significance and value. If this is important to you, make the commitment to write down what you're doing. You'll see your progress as you gain fitness and endurance, and you'll eventually amaze yourself with the cumulative total of the hours and miles you put in.

You can do your log however you want. High-tech versions include software that lets you enter all your planned and actual workouts, graph them in a variety of ways, publish them to the Web, and upload data from your heart-rate monitor or bike computer. This may appeal to you. Other people might prefer a spiral-bound notebook and a Bic pen. There are also some Web sites that allow you to enter your data online, either free or for a subscription fee. These are cool but they never let you enter all the data you want in the form that you want. My coach has just started using www.trainingbible.com, and that's pretty handy. I used to use an Excel spreadsheet. Some people scrawl their workouts on a calendar. You can buy books like *The Triathlete's Training Diary For Dummies* or the *Inside Triathlon Training Diary*. So you have a lot of options.

The basics you would want to record are when, what, how long, how hard, and how you feel. You might want to put in how sore you are when you get up in the morning, with 1 being fresh as the proverbial daisy and 10 being "Wild buffalo have stampeded over my entire body." Rate the quality of your sleep likewise, with 1 being the best and 10 being nasty insomnia. Fatigue, same thing. And then your overall well-being. Is it a pretty good day?

It might look like this:

Sample Training Log

Date	Workout	Time	Distance	Soreness (1-10)	Sleep (1-10)	Tiredness (1-10)	Overall (1-10)	Notes
5/5/04	Bike	1:30	20.4	3	3	3	4	moderate cruise
5/6/04	Run	:44	4	2	6	7	6	ez warm-up, 20-min. tempo, cool down
5/6/04	Swim	:30	.5	4	3	4	5	800 yards

Over time, you'll start to see patterns and progress that will maybe help you to avoid getting overtired or help you figure out when you have your best workouts.

Enough with these preliminaries—let's get you in the pool.

SWIMMING

FOR MANY PEOPLE, getting to the pool is the biggest obstacle to doing a tri. You actually have to go somewhere just to get started, it's inconvenient, it's chlorinated, and you have to change into a bathing suit in front of other people. But once you find a congenial pool setting and get in the habit of going, it can be very soothing. I've always loved water, and I find the feel of it on my skin and the sound of my walrus-like breathing as I inch along my lane to induce a calming, meditative state. This may be one of the reasons why I have such a hard time swimming fast. I mean, I'm lying down and cool water is flowing over me. I feel much more like sleeping than going hard. But enough about me for a while. Where are you going to swim?

Depending on where you live, you may have an overwhelming number of options or you may have almost none. My friend Michelle wanted her Mom to go to water aerobics classes for her rheumatoid arthritis symptoms, but the nearest pool to Mom's home in Odum, Georgia, was almost an hour's drive away. Mrs. Oakes's second option was to swim in the pond on the farm, but the water moccasins had other ideas. Odum is pretty darn rural though, so hopefully you can find somewhere to swim pretty near your house. If you've managed to locate a triathlon club in your area, ask around for good swimming options. As a conversational opener for triathletes, I find that "So, where do you swim?" is almost as good as the weather.

Some people like the comfort and convenience of health clubs. Others opt to save money and buy a pass to the city pool. I chose a middle ground with a YMCA membership. A lot of folks who are serious about improving their swimming sign up for Masters' swimming clubs. I was kind of confused when I heard about Masters'—I thought it meant that you had to be good at swimming. But no, all it means is that you're over eighteen and have a strong masochistic streak. Masters' workouts have set hours, coaches, and structure. The coaches usually put people in lanes based on their pace, so the faster people and the slower folks don't bump into each other.

I've been swimming for about three years now and I still haven't taken the step of attending Masters' workouts. I think they're terrific for improving your swimming. It's just that I pay money to the YMCA every month, so I figure I should use their pool. The Y also has a Masters' club, but I just stubbornly go and swim by myself. Part of this is also my unwillingness to have too many strictly scheduled workout times. However, in another shining example of not practicing what I preach, I'm going to tell you that structured workouts of one kind or another are a fantastic tool for triathletes. When I have participated in them, they've been incredibly helpful. They build camaraderie and help get you motivated to get up and get out there with your buddies. You probably need to feel pretty comfortable in the pool and be able to swim a good few laps of the pool to get the most out of Masters' workouts. If you are confident that you can go up and back a few times without passing out, and you like the idea of suffering in company with others, by all means contact the local Masters' club.

A lot of first-time triathletes (and even twentieth-time triathletes) dread the swim part of the event. In fact, let me back way up to step one. Can you swim? Because if you can't, that does pose a bit of an obstacle to completing a triathlon. Not an insurmountable one, but something that would need to be addressed sooner rather than later. A lot of communities teach adult swim lessons through their Parks or Recreation Department, offering a safe, low-key place to get your feet wet, and then work up to the rest of you. You'll want to focus on your freestyle stroke, but definitely enjoy the other ways of getting through the water, like breaststroke and backstroke. They can come in handy even in a race, if you want to just take a break from crawling along face down. My coach was just telling me about a client of hers who had never done any swimming, but wanted to train for and complete a triathlon. She was also totally freaked out about water that she couldn't see the bottom of. But she did the training and did the race, doing the breaststroke the entire swim.

The point is, as my point always is, just get your bad self in the water and swim. Doggie paddle or do the Esther Williams sidestroke if you want. No, I'm not old enough to remember Esther Williams, but I've seen clips of those MGM musicals of the '30s and '40s, and she looked really elegant gliding through the water on her side. I did an open water race last year where one guy swam the 2.4-mile course using nothing but butterfly. That's the one where you fling both arms out of the water at the same time while simultaneously making your lower body do dolphin-like things. I do two strokes of butterfly and I feel like I'm gonna need shoulder surgery. Different strokes, as they say.

So if you're starting from absolute square one, can't swim a stroke, I would add a few months onto your timeline for getting race-ready. Even if you pick up the swimming part really quickly, you want to feel good and comfortable in the water before you get into that open water, group swimming situation.

If you can already knock out a couple hundred yards or more of freestyle, your task is easier. Say your first sprint distance triathlon has a four-hundred-yard swim leg. That's sixteen lengths of a twenty-five-yard pool. Even if you can only do one or two lengths consecutively now, you can tack on twenty-five yards each workout and be up to distance within a couple of months. Get out a piece of paper and write down what your swimming capacity is now—how long can you swim without stopping and without getting exhausted? How much distance can you cover in that time? If you have no idea, use your first session in the pool to establish a baseline. How comfortable do you feel in a pool? Rate your comfort level on a scale of 1 to 5, with 1 being "Totally Relaxed, Pass the Margaritas" and 5 being, "Please God, Don't Make Me Put My Face in the Water, *no, no, no!*"

Use this rudimentary evaluation to set some goals. Besides your goal of completing your race, insert some stepping-stone goals. If you can do one hundred yards now, set goals of getting up to two hundred yards and then three hundred in a session. If your race is four hundred, I would also set a goal of being able to swim significantly longer than four hundred without a break. Maybe say eight hundred yards, or at least six hundred. It might seem like a lot now, but you'll work up to it pretty quick, and you'll feel much more confident when you step into the water on race day, knowing that the swim distance is not a problem for you.

TECHNIQUE

I'm not going to tell you how to improve your stroke because I know almost nothing about swimming. I recently paid a swim coach fifty bucks to analyze my stroke and videotape me underwater, and boy, was that a jolting experience. It turns out I was doing some of the most fundamental things absolutely wrong. I was dropping my elbows, pulling to the side, not kicking enough, taking too few strokes—a nightmare! It's amazing I was able to get from one side of the pool to the other. On the other hand, I have quite a significant amount of natural flotation in the form of body fat, so that helps keep me positioned high in the water. But I digress.

What I *am* going to tell you is that technique is more important in swimming than cycling or running, because the effect of drag in the water is so intense. You can get much faster for less energy expenditure if you make your stroke more efficient and your body more streamlined in the water. So take advantage of every opportunity you can to improve your stroke technique. A book that at least got me part of the way there is *Swimming Made Easy* by Terry Laughlin. He also has a Web site where you can buy videos, sign up for clinics for his Total Immersion swimming instruction, and pick up other books.

THE DEVIL AND THE DEEP BLUE SEA

Some triathlons do have a swim leg that takes place in a pool. Most of them, though, including the really fun ones, make you get out into the open water. No lane marker, no black line on the bottom; in fact, you can't even see the bottom. The water might be cold, there might be slimy weeds or fish in it, or even jellyfish if you've got an ocean swim. And of course (low, menacing bass music) . . . sharks. If you grew up with *Jaws* and its progeny, no amount of rationalizing about the minuscule chances of getting attacked by a shark while doing a triathlon is going to make you any less convinced that gory death awaits you when you're out there far from shore. Better just to put it out of your mind completely. Yeah, easy for me to say, I know. I confess, I have had some ocean swims where I couldn't quite stop imagining what might be swimming around below me, looking up at me through pitiless, black, gleaming eyes. But remember, your chances of getting hurt in a car crash on the way to the ocean are so much greater.

Seriously, folks, it's a good idea to practice open water swimming before your first race. It's a different animal altogether. If you can find a local club, chances are there'll be some organized open water sessions at some point in the season. Definitely check it out. You might contact local swimming organizations, but mostly they stick to that wimpy pool stuff. Triathletes are kind of in the forefront of open water swimming. Or you could find a public beach or lake or whatever kind of waterway you have in your parts. Take someone with you who knows what they're doing and can coach you through the swim. Find a landmark on shore, or a buoy or boat in the water, and practice sighting it as you swim, lifting your head quickly every five to ten strokes or so. Work on keeping a straight line. If you're going to use a wetsuit in the race, use a wetsuit in your practice swims so you get used to the feel of that clingy rubber around your limbs.

CYCLING

YOU CAN DO this. It's just like riding a bike. But now you're In Training for a Triathlon, so it becomes cycling instead. The major logistical challenges in training yourself for the bike leg are finding more or less safe roads to train on and enough daylight to train in. If you live in Boston, you will be forced to drive with your bike at least twenty miles to get out of the homicidal reach of Boston's maniacal drivers. (Sorry, the scars from my pedestrian college years in Beantown haven't fully healed. More therapy is in order.) You may be lucky enough to live in an area with bike trails, or quiet winding roads with wide shoulders. If you're just starting out, you can probably do your whole workout on a ten-mile bike trail. At the very least, look for roads with wide shoulders or wide right lanes, relatively light traffic, and not too many traffic lights.

If you're having trouble thinking of a good bike route where you live, contact your local cycling club or bike store. Use the Web to search for bike routes. It took me less than five minutes just now to find five Web pages with information on rides around Columbia, South Carolina. In fact, I know where to meet the weekly summer riding groups, how fast they go, how far they go, and that one of the rides is a community service trash pickup ride.

Here's another "Do as I say, not as I do" (DAIS, NAID) piece of advice—ride with other people. This way, if one of you has a fall or a mechanical problem that you can't fix, you've got someone there to help you out. If you can't do this because of your schedule or your skulking loner personality, carry a cell phone and ID. That way the folks who come to scrape you off the pavement will at least know who you are. I like to ride by myself most of the time, but the area I live in is pretty densely populated and simply crawling with cyclists on all the good routes, so I never feel truly alone.

Use common sense to avoid having to be scraped off the pavement in the first place. Assume cars can't see you at all as you ride along, even though you're wearing your gaudiest gold, red, and green jersey for visibility. Ride as far to the right as is practicable. Keep in a straight line and don't do anything unpredictable if you can help it. Don't run red lights or stop signs (again, DAIS, NAID) because intersections are where most car-bike accidents happen. If you do ride with other people, ride in single file. Nothing irks me more in cyclists than seeing riders cruising along four abreast, chatting about the latest race wheels. They may be making a statement about having just as much right to the lane as a semi or a Ford Exterminator, but get real, boys and girls! Even a tiny car can crush your ass! Get your butt out of the way and live to ride another day. Keep alert for potholes, storm gratings, road debris, and especially—the cyclist's nightmare—a car door opening in front of you as you zoom down the right-hand side of the road.

And do I really have to tell you to wear a helmet every single time you get on a bicycle for any distance whatsoever?

Having said all that and frightened the Lycra cycling pants off you, I want to tell you that cycling is also fun. It's not just a white-knuckle suicide run among crazy drivers and road hazards. It's being outside, feeling the wind on your face and the road rushing under your wheels. It's swooping around a big corner and testing the conservation of angular momentum, or looking up and seeing a hawk on a telephone pole. It's smelling the damp earth and new grass after a spring rain or the tantalizing aromas of the neighborhood's dinners as you ride home at dusk. You can go as far as your legs can take you, and it's free.

Now get your piece of paper that you used for your swimming self-assessment, and prepare to do the same thing for cycling. What's a comfortable amount of time for you to ride? How far do you get in that time? If you don't have a bike computer, you can drive around your bike route and check mileage on your car odometer. How comfortable do you feel on a bike? What things are hard for you? Uphills? Downhills? Riding in traffic? Now, where do you want to be by race day, or by the end of the summer, or the end of the year? Just like swimming, pick some milestones along the way that are significant but achievable. Find a hill that looks like a good intermediate goal, or a distance that's further than you can ride right now. Just like with swimming, I recommend training yourself up to a distance beyond what you will have to ride in a race. It just gives you that extra little security blanket, knowing that you've done the extra work ahead of time.

If you're one of those people whose life is defined by their job, you leave your house in the pre-dawn gloom and don't return until dark and all that crap, it might be tough for you to schedule a safe time to ride. My advice is to restructure your life so that your work is either a lower priority or a shorter commute. OK, got that handled? All right, all right, so some people do have legitimate reasons for their four-hour commutes and twelve-hour days. But why'd you pick up this book if you didn't have at least some theoretical interest in trying something different? Maybe the something different is getting your work schedule trimmed down a little so you can get outside and work toward a triathlon. I just feel like one of the biggest flaws in American life is that we think we are what we do for a living. "Senior Project Manager—It's Not Just a Job, It's My Identity." You're so much more than that. And there's even a slow fat triathlete inside you, waiting to come out.

If you work long hours and can't get out on the road during the week, or if you live in a place with abysmal weather, try an indoor cycling class at the city recreation department or your local gym. Those classes can whip you into shape in a hurry, and the cool thing is that you're not going to get nine miles out on the road and realize you're too pooped to get home. Get out on the road at least once on the weekend though—it helps to actually ride the bike, steering, braking, all that stuff. And here's another little secret—some people only ride once a week and still do triathlons.

Oh, and please do learn to fix a flat. It is so annoying to get outside on a gorgeous spring day and then have to call your spouse. "Honey, there's no air in my tire. What'll I do? Can you come get me, please? Pleeeeeaze?" It's just too whiney for words. Tire irons, a spare tube, a patch kit, and a pump that fits on your bike. Don't leave home without 'em. The bike shop will give you instructions on how to do it if you ask nicely.

RUNNING

LOGISTICALLY, THIS IS probably the easiest sport to train yourself to do. Just put on your shoes and head out the door. However, it's probably the easiest sport to injure yourself in, so I repeat all my admonitions to go easy, easy, easy on yourself, wear good shoes, take little strides, and stay relaxed. This is also the sport that gets your heart rate up the highest, too, so if you have any cardiac risk factors, again, check with the friendly doc. If you get any twinges in your legs or feet when you run, stop and go home. Put an ice pack on the twinge-y bit for twenty minutes when you get home, and take your over-the-counter painkiller of choice. (Lots of athletes swear by Advil for the aches and pains, but I find it burns a fiery hole in my stomach. Likewise Aleve, the panacea of many endurance athletes. I stick to aspirin.) And then go real easy on the sore part of you. Don't even contemplate running while you still feel pain. On your next run, if you feel the same pain again, stop, do not pass Go, return to home base, and await instructions from the mother ship. And the mother ship will say, "Ice some more, more painkillers, rest some more."

If this keeps up for more than a few days, go get it checked out with your doctor. You may have some issues with your muscles, joints, cartilage, whatever. You may have funky-shaped feet that need extra support in the form of stabilizing running shoes or even orthotics. Or you may just be taking it too fast.

You also want to keep your personal safety in mind, of course. If you're a woman, you're probably more aware of safety issues than I am—I live in a pretty harmless area, I'm big and strong, and I stubbornly refuse to believe that running at 7 P.M. in a suburban neighborhood is going to put me in grave danger. But I know most of my friends are more sensible than I am. They run with other friends and Rottweilers and carry pepper spray and all that. Use your common sense and your intuition and (DAIS, NAID) err on the side of caution.

If you're already a runner of even modest ability and experience, I would definitely recommend hooking up with some kind of coached running workout as soon as possible. If there's a triathlon club or running club in your area that offers access to a coached track or running session, put your head up, firmly suppress your anxieties and insecurities, and go check it out. I spent a lot of time being the very last person to finish track workouts, but I've gotten a little faster and learned a lot about pacing, effort, and good running technique from doing it.

Once again, get out your grimy little piece of paper and do a self-evaluation on your current level of running preparedness. Can you jog even a little bit? How long can you jog before hailing the nearest cab? Do you know how much ground you can cover in that time? Do you have any medical conditions that you need to get checked out before you even put running shoe to pavement? Figure out the small steps you need to take so that you can work up to the running leg of the triathlon.

One great resource for building up your running is the Couch-to-5K Running Plan at www.coolrunning.com. It's got a detailed eight-week plan outlining each workout, how much warm-up time to include, how long to jog and how long to walk each time, and some good stuff about stretching and staying loose. I know lots of people online who have moved from couch spuds to confident 5K runners using this exact plan, and it's really similar to how I get myself back in shape to run. Runner's World online (www.runnersworld.com) also has a good section for new runners and a great article on walking/running as an excellent way to train, not just for beginners, but for all of us.

YOU DON'T EVEN HAVE TO RUN

It's true—you don't have to run if you don't want to. If you have orthopedic issues or severe anxiety about running, you can certainly complete a triathlon by walking the run leg. I've seen it done, and nothing indicated to me that those finishers had any less fun than the faster folks. In fact, you don't ever have to run if you don't want to. Just getting out of your door a few times a week and working your way gradually up to walking a couple of miles is an achievement in my book.

If you do want to make an attempt at running, the jog-walk combination is an incredibly powerful tool for sofa-dwellers aspiring to raise their level of athleticism. Jog for thirty seconds, walk for thirty seconds. Repeat for twenty minutes. If you can't keep that up for twenty minutes, then jog for fifteen seconds and walk for a minute. Whatever it takes. Start where you are right now—don't try and skip a step—and just work your way gradually up to where you can jog for twenty minutes without walking. At that point you'll probably be up to about 1.7 to 1.9 miles for that twenty minutes. You're two thirds of the way there if your first race has a 5K or 3.1-mile run. And don't hesitate to take walk breaks in training or racing whenever you feel that you need them. There's a whole school of distance runners out there who take planned walk breaks every ten minutes or so, and use this technique to complete marathons in eminently respectable times—between three and three-and-a-half hours, which I can only dream of. Use the "talk test" to see if you're working too hard: If you can't carry on a conversation with your running buddy or with the empty air, you ought to slow down a little.

STRETCHING

STRETCHING IS THE too-often overlooked fourth discipline of triathlon training. Stretching regularly and patiently can reduce your risk of injury, improve your performance, and make you feel a lot less decrepit after a workout. The key areas to look out for as a triathlete are

- Calves
- Quads
- Hamstrings
- Glutes
- Lower Back
- Groin
- Shoulders
- Neck

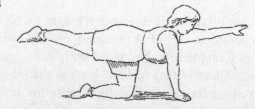

If you have some background in how to stretch these body bits safely, then please just do so after your workouts. If you have no idea where your glutes or quads are, then do me a favor and sign up for a stretching class at the community center, or, at the very least, buy a book or video on stretching. I could do a whole chapter just on stretching, but it's not really what I'm here for. What I do want to say is that when I neglect my stretching, that's when I get hurt. All the leg stretches help to keep your legs and hips loose, mobile, and properly aligned, and that in turn helps take strain off your back. When I don't stretch, I hurt my back, and then I'm out of training for anywhere from one to four weeks. I've done this three times now, and each time I'm hurt, I get right back on the floor and work on my stretching. The pain goes away, and eventually my stretching routine does, too. Then I get hurt again. So (all together now) *"Do as I say, not as I do!"* Stretch after every workout. This is the most effective time to do it. Your muscles are warm and loose from the exercise, and you can gently get them to lengthen a little as they cool down. If you stretch before a workout, that's not a terrible thing, but your muscles are cold and not too flexible then, so be extra slow, careful, and patient. You're better off warming up very slowly as part of your workout and stretching afterwards.

Build a base in all three disciplines. Get to the point where you can do your target distances comfortably and you stretch with religious devotion. Then, a few weeks before race time, or earlier if you want, start preparing yourself for transitions.

TRANSITIONS

DID SOMEONE SAY triathlon was swimming, cycling, and running? Oh, was that me? Well, I misspoke. Stretching is the fourth discipline, and transitions are the fifth. Or the other way round. Anyway, you have to do transitions if you're going to be in a race, and it's kind of fun to take some time to practice them. A lot of people don't, especially before their first race, but I found a little transition practice was really helpful in a couple of respects. First off, I knew what to expect and it helped me to be calmer and more cheerful on race morning. Secondly, it helped me to be faster, and any time that I could make up without having to actually be out on the course gaining on someone is like a special free gift.

Maybe you've decided you're just going to do your first race for pure fun and just to finish and you don't care about your time at all. That's cool. Just humor me and read these next couple paragraphs, so at least they'll be in the back of your mind come race day.

There are only two transitions you have to worry about. We call them T1 (swim to bike) and T2 (bike to run). Come closer, grasshopper. Transition practice is your stealth weapon.

Before you even have a transition, you have set-up. A key to having a fast transition and less stress in your race is having your gear set up in a way that makes sense for you. You'll put your bike on the bike rack, and then you'll have a couple feet of space between you and the next person's bike where you have to fit your helmet, your bike shoes, sunglasses, running shoes, hat, extra water, and whatever else you might want. The way almost all triathlons work is that you start and finish very close to the transition area. So you set up your stuff, and you go walk a couple hundred yards to the swim start. When you're done swimming, you run back to transition, make yourself into a cyclist, and pedal away. You finish cycling back at the transition area. You leave your bike at your spot on the rack, transform into a runner, and head off again. Then you run back to the finish, which is probably less than a couple hundred yards from the transition area where you left your bike. There are some races that don't follow this pattern, but they're pretty few and far between. We're going to base our transition lessons on having one transition area, to which you will keep returning like a swallow in the spring.

So, first thing we practice is set-up. First, position your bike on something that can serve as a rack. Face the bike toward you, so that the front wheel and handlebars are closest to you when you come running up from the swim. Now, take a smallish towel or a folded big towel and put it next to your bike. The towel is handy to mark out territory and to wipe your feet on after the swim. Make it as gaudy and eye-catching as possible. This will help you find your bike among the hundreds of other bikes in the transition area. Put your bike helmet, shoes and socks, and other bike accessories (sunglasses, gloves) on the towel in a position where they'll be easy to reach as you come in. Then take your running shoes and anything else you'll have on the run (cap, race number belt) and put them out on the towel, too. OK, now we may proceed.

T1—SWIM TO BIKE

If you can practice the transition from swim to bike coming out of open water with your wetsuit on, that would be the ideal scenario. Have a supportive friend or spouse watch your bike and run gear while you swim around a little, then come charging out of the water. Swim long enough to get a good sense of what it's like to shift from horizontal swimmer to vertical runner. One tip that comes straight from the pros is to swim as long as you can until your hand hits bottom. If you stand up when the water is chest deep, you're going to expend a ton of extra energy flailing through the water to the shore.

And look out when you do get back onto solid ground. One thing that no triathlon book or fellow triathlete warned me about is that when you get out of the water, you will probably feel dizzy. Something to do with the middle ear and the horizontal position and the cold water and other technical things. When I went out to practice my T1 for the first time, I couldn't believe how hard it was just to jog in a straight line. I felt like I had just had two shots of vodka and a tank full of laughing gas. And to this day I sometimes have to sit down to finish pulling my wetsuit off and get my bike shoes on. Some triathletes have less sensitive inner ears, more practice, or better coordination than I (probably all of the above) and manage to stand on one leg to get the wetsuit around their ankles.

Pulling the wetsuit off is the biggest challenge in all of triathlon. It's also really hard to describe how to do it efficiently. The basic idea is to start getting the thing off quickly, while it's still holding enough water to be somewhat forgiving. (The more it dries out, the less stretchy it is.) Reach behind your back, grab your zipper pull, yank it down, and wriggle out of the top half. This will be much harder than it sounds because you'll be trying to jog forward as you do this and your arms will have all the strength of a campaign promise. Then run run run back to your transition area with your wetsuit sleeves flapping around you. When you get there, yank the suit down over your behind and then roll it off your legs like you're peeling a banana. Don't push the legs down in a bunch. This is a recipe for falling over and causing unrestrained spectator amusement. Pull your feet out with conviction, quickly place the suit somewhere it won't get too thrashed by the mob, and quick-change into a cyclist. Don't bother drying off or anything. Just go.

You have to have your helmet on and clipped before you move your bike anywhere. It's the rules. So get it on, grab your shades, don't stab yourself in the face with them like I do, and put your shoes on as fast as you know how. Practice putting your shoes on fast, whatever kind of shoes you use. Socks are optional. For short races, you may not need them at all. On the other hand, if you're more comfortable with socks, take the twenty seconds to put them on. But practice putting them on fast. Unless of course your race time means nothing to you, in which case, sit back, file your foot calluses, touch up your toenail polish, and then put your socks and shoes on in as leisurely a manner as you want to. It's fine with me, especially if you're racing in my age group. If you use gloves, put them on now or Velcro them around your handlebars and put them on as you ride. For a short race, you might not want them.

OK, now you've got your cycling gear on. Grab your bike off the rack and trot to the bike exit. You remember where the bike exit is from your pre-race scouting, right? Watch and listen to the volunteers who will tell you when you can get on your bike. When the moment is right, get on the bike and pedal smoothly away. D'oh! You left your bike in the hardest gear and you can't move your legs! Avoid this common yet spectator-amusing mistake—make sure the bike is in a medium-low gear when you rack it up.

And there you are—on the bike leg! You would not believe how much more relaxed you will feel on race day knowing that you have practiced this transition and have a small clue about what you're going to do in what order. Now, what happens when you come in off the bike?

T2–BIKE TO RUN

This one's a lot simpler, but you can still benefit from a few repetitions beforehand. Cruise in on your bike and dismount before the dismount line. In a race, you should be able to tell where the dismount line is because volunteers will be screaming at you to slow down and get off the bike. If you're practicing, make up a dismount line about twenty-five yards from your practice transition area, and get off there. Run with your bike to your rack and hang the bike up by the handlebars this time. Off with the helmet, off with the shoes, on with the running shoes, and you're done. As I head out, I grab a mesh running cap to protect my tender nose from the sun. I also put my race number on a little elastic belt, so I grab that too and put it on as I run out. If you have your number safety-pinned to your race shirt, you're all set. I have an issue with sharp pointy things and try to avoid situations where they might be close to my body in any way because I'm a great big klutz. But that's me.

The other thing to practice about T2 is just the motion of running after cycling. Your legs will most likely feel like alien appendages made from an amalgam of lead and rubber. It will just feel wrong to run. This is normal. And you can definitely train your legs to get used to that feeling and run through it. After a while you do get your regular legs back. If your regular legs aren't trained well for the run, they might not feel good, but they will at least be your legs.

THE BRICK WORKOUT–FOUNDATION OF TRIATHLON PREPAREDNESS

To prepare for the run off the bike, practice it. Go for a bike ride, then go for a run right afterwards. This is called a "brick" in triathlon parlance. You can do a swim-bike brick or a bike-run brick. The bike-run is more useful. When you do your first brick, take a short, easy ride, then do a short, easy run. Next time, do a normal bike ride, then a short easy run. If your first race is a sprint distance, get yourself to the point where you can do a brick that's your whole bike distance and your whole run distance. You don't have to do this, but then again it'll make you feel mighty and confident on race day.

You can also practice a swim-bike brick, just for kicks. The easiest way is to bring your bike to your open water swim and hop on it as soon as you're done swimming. Don't even towel off—just put your shoes and helmet on and go. This will get you used to the unusual sensation of riding along all dripping wet and soggy.

Brick workouts are the best time to figure out what's going to work for you in your clothing selection. For both kinds of bricks, wear the clothes you plan to wear on race day. If you plan to race in your bike shorts, the brick may bring you the unwelcome news that running in your bike shorts is like trying to run wearing Pampers. Or it might work just fine. If you're brave enough to wear a swimsuit for the whole race, make sure that running and cycling in it doesn't lead to nasty chafing.

BUT WHATEVER SHALL I WEAR?

AS YOUR TRAINING builds up to race day, you will start to turn your attention to other matters, like your racing wardrobe. I find that a lot of us beginning triathletes don't have the kind of positive body image that allows us to compete in just a bathing suit, so then you have to be creative and balance out your need for coverage with your need for speed and comfort. If you'll hark back to Chapter Three, you'll remember a rather heated diatribe against training in cotton. This goes double for racing. To recap: Cotton gets wet and stays wet. It gets heavy. It can chafe, and you can get chilled racing in it when it's wet.

When you're looking for speed in transitions and good functionality, you want to look at changing clothes as few times as possible. Preferably none. I wear exactly what I'm going to wear for the bike and the run under my wetsuit. That would be my bomb-proof sports bra, my figure-hugging tri top, and my lightly padded tri shorts. If I was doing a non-wetsuit swim, I'd have to experiment a little. I might swim in the sleeveless tri top, or I might just swim in the sports bra and tug the top on after the swim. The trade off is that you either lose time in the water from the drag of the top, or lose time in transition trying to squirm a wet body into a tight-fitting garment. I haven't raced in any warm water yet, so it's all hypothetical for me.

If you're a woman who's built smaller than I am, you can swim, bike, and run in either a sports bra or a workout top with a built-in bra. For me, those little tops or shimmels (why *are* they called that?) just don't provide anywhere near the level of support I need for running. And there's no way in hell I'm running around in public in just my sports bra. It's that body image thing.

If you're a boy, breast support shouldn't be an issue, even if you do have some extra tissue in the pectoral area. You can swim in your tri shorts and your top for a wetsuit race, or tuck your tri top down into your shorts for a non-wetsuit race and pull it up over your shoulders as you come out of the water.

Or you can take your time in transition and put a nice baggy non-cotton T-shirt on over whatever you swam in. It'll cover up your love handles, but it'll flap around on the bike. No big deal. Note for boys— you may want to look into putting band-aids over your nipples. Seriously. Remember, the slow fat triathlete is an expert on chafe-avoidance.

Figure out what you want from the race and then plan accordingly. If one of the fun parts of the game for you is figuring out how to shave a few seconds in transition, plan your clothing strategy accordingly and then practice it. If you're just going out to participate and have fun, then take your fluffy towels and your battery-powered hairdryer and take it easy in transition. The important thing is that you're out there.

TRAINED AND READY

FAST FORWARD TO a couple of weeks before your target race. Depending on what you've done with your time, you should feel reasonably ready to strap it on come race day and have a good time. You have your equipment in order. You know what you're going to wear. You know you can do the distance. You're ready. You've trained. You are strong like an Amazon. Or like the Terminator. Whatever rings your chimes.

And if you're not, for whatever reason, please consider withdrawing from the race. If your training didn't come together, if you got injured or you lost steam, it's better to pull out of a race than to get injured. Again, all together now, "Do as I say . . ." There will be other races, but injuries are painful, frustrating, and boring.

If you're ready to rrrrrummmmmbblllllle, go ahead and move on to the next chapter. If you feel like reading about one of the training adventures that helped make my 2003 season so much fun, check out the following.

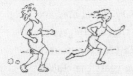

Training Days
April 14, 2003

I was reading back over my collection of race reports, and I realized that they mostly focus on the dramas, embarrassments, and glories of race day itself, maybe a little bit about the day before. And that is such a tiny part of the triathlon life. I spent something like twelve hours racing in triathlons last season and hundreds of hours preparing for those twelve hours. Between the training, the bike maintenance, and the hours spent drooling over equipment catalogues and tri Web sites, it sucks up a lot of time. So I thought I'd try and share a little about what it's like.

The day-in, day-out training blurs together most of the time. Up until a few weeks ago, I followed a fairly flexible schedule. I just tried to get three runs, two swims and two bike workouts into my week. And a lot of the time in the off-season I'd settle for one swim and one bike. I'd try to go to club track sessions every Tuesday night to run intervals and otherwise suffer in the name of gaining some foot speed. And starting each January, there's the club's New to the Sport program, which offers coached Saturday rides and Sunday runs. So I tagged along with those workouts and invented a few of my own and managed to get fitter and a little faster.

Then I temporarily took leave of my senses and signed up for a half-Ironman race in September. When I returned to the home planet, I was scared witless. I had no idea how I was going to get my creaky bod to that level of endurance. Rule of thumb in triathlon—when in doubt, spend some more money. So I hired a coach. Lisa, who coaches our track sessions on Tuesdays, had already worked wonders for several other club members, so I winced and wrote out a fat check entitling me to personalized training plans, extra track practice, and lots of good advice.

Now things are a lot more structured. I have leeway to figure out my own schedule, but there's a lot of stuff that has to fit into a week, and one day has to be scheduled as an off day. Monday swim, Tuesday swim and track practice, Wednesday bike, Thursday track and/or yoga, Friday swim, Saturday bike, Sunday run. Oops, no rest day that way. Try scheduling it again. OK, Monday off, put a swim and a bike on Wednesday. Yup, that ought to do it. Then I just have to make sure that I don't do speed or hill work in cycling and running on the same day. I need project management software just to handle my hobby.

In between times there's trying to squeeze in a few stretches on the floor in front of the TV, or spending some intense sessions working on transition skills.

The weeks pretty much whiz by in a tornado of sweaty sports bras and moist bathing suits. Every so often there's a training session that really gets everyone's attention: a group open water swim, a crazy Santa Cruz Mountain Bike ride, a trail run on someone's wedding day. The last two years the club's Wildflower training camp weekend has been the most epic of these. It's a great opportunity to get together with fellow club members, camp out in a beautiful spot, and practice running and riding up and down the endless hills surrounding Lake San Antonio. Lots of hanging out and a big ol' barbecue dinner, and the chance to talk to the athletes I never get to see because they're always running twice as fast as I am.

So last Saturday I got up at 5:15 in the morning and packed all my junk in the car for the two-and-a-half-hour drive down to the lake. The wind was howling and the rain started coming down in Mountain View just as I was loading the car.

It wasn't yet raining (much) at the lake, so I was able to get my tent set up on dry, almost level ground. We got together in a huge mob and set off on the bike ride in an obnoxious wind. "This is pretty much just going to suck," I thought to myself, and in fact I voiced this thought aloud to anyone who would listen. It did. The 24.8-mile Olympic distance course took me about 1:50 to complete, which is pretty slow for me, as the bike is my strongest leg. Strong cold winds, brisk rain showers, and some nasty hills. The long-course riders had fifty-six miles of this fun, even more wind, even more hills.

It started raining in earnest just before dinner on Saturday evening, though we stayed cheerful while we were being fed huge chunks of marinated tri tip and while the campfire blazed. I silently thanked L.L. Bean for my rain pants. It rained all night and was still raining pretty hard on Sunday morning. I stayed fairly dry in my tent, but it was hard to sleep through the noise of the rain. I was surrounded by evil pixies popping endless sheets of bubble wrap right next to my ear until it was light enough to get up.

When I finally dragged myself out into the moist morning air, people were packing up and bailing left and right. But peer pressure induced about twenty of us to get our wetsuits on and go for a brisk swim around the houseboats. This proved to be a capital idea as we were warmer and drier in our wetsuits than we had been at any time that weekend.

The swim was another insane opportunity to develop mental toughness—there was some pretty stiff chop on the lake and swimming into the wind made the water feel like Jell-O. Once that was done I was just eager to get packed, get dry, and get home. I wore my wetsuit to break camp, slithering around in the oak forest like a giant black slug. I got some semi-dry clothes on in the restroom and bolted for home, abandoning my plan to tackle the Wildflower run course and promising myself an easy run after I got home and unpacked.

Ha. I was so exhausted when I got home and got all my wet stuff out onto the patio to dry that all I could do was pass out on the couch. I slept through the final thrilling minutes of the Paris-Roubaix bike race, which just shows you how tired I was.

So I don't know what exactly to think about my preparedness for the race. The abysmal conditions made everything hard to judge. In fact, they made everything just plain hard. I can tell I'm not going to set a personal record on either the bike or the run, but I have no idea how bad it's going to be. All I know is it's not going to be fifty-five degrees and raining with twenty-mile-per-headwinds on the day. Nothing for it but to jump back into the routine. Monday swim, Tuesday track, Wednesday swim and bike, and see what happens on race day.

And that's fine. Because the moment of truth isn't when you line up at the start and peer out into the water with your heart pounding with fear and excitement, and it's not when you drag your quivering limbs across the finish line. I mean, those are moments of truth, but they're just two moments among so many more. Every time you stuff your suit and goggles into your fraying gym bag for the lunchtime swim; every time you change in the office bathroom on your way to track; every time you show up at the bike shop for that quad-busting Saturday ride—they're all moments of truth. And all the little moments of truth end up adding up to some larger aggregate truth. The real fun is figuring out what that is.

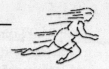

The Slow Fat Triathlete
Recommends

This was a really long chapter, and it was pretty much all practical advice, but I'm going to give you the cheat sheet right here so that training stays (or becomes) enjoyable for you and deposits you on race day feeling happy and confident, underneath all your superficial nervousness.

1. Be really smart about any medical stuff you may have going on. If you've been diagnosed with hypertension, or high cholesterol, or you've smoked for thirty years, you need to check in with the medical folks to work out a gradual way to work into exercise.

2. Even if you're basically "presumed healthy," start slow, and keep going slow for way longer than you think you have to. This is true of each individual workout, and it's true of your training program in general. Six weeks of easing into your workout schedule is probably the minimum if you aren't already exercising.

3. Be realistic about who you are and what you can do right now. There may be no limit to what you can do with patience and training, but do a really hard-headed assessment of what you can do right now. I hate to generalize, but I will anyway: I think guys are more prone to overestimating their current fitness than women are. I think a lot of women, especially those no longer in their first blush of youth, think, "Oh, I can't do that." Then they get to surprise themselves in a good way.

4. Find a training schedule that works for you. If you need to get to work earlier so that you can leave earlier and ride your bike, see if you can arrange that flexibility with your boss. If you can't work out six days a week, don't. Do what you can do, and if you really like it, you'll find ways to make more time for it.

5. It's way better to do a little bit consistently than to do a big workout, then skip a few days, then do another big workout. If you can get out and jog for twenty minutes, do it. Don't wait until you can get out for forty minutes.

6. And you know, this stuff works for everyone—not just triathletes. Most of us could use the mental and physical benefits of more exercise. If your goal isn't doing a triathlon, set some other goal. Tell yourself you're going to walk to the coffee shop five miles away by the time fall comes. You can take a cab home or call your honey for a ride. Just make it a priority to move your butt at whatever level you can.

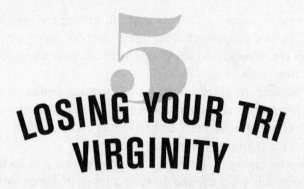

LOSING YOUR TRI VIRGINITY

HOW TO HAVE FUN
YOUR VERY FIRST TIME

WOW, CHECK YOU out, girlfriend! And guys, too! Y'all are the bomb! You're all that and a bag of chips! You are ready for race day, dudes and dudettes! You have found equipment, you've put in your hours of preparation in the pool and on the road, and somewhere real soon, that moment of truth is lurking on your horizon. But remember from the last chapter that every moment is a moment of truth, and don't be intimidated by what you've set out to do.

THE WEEK BEFORE

WITH SEVEN DAYS to go before race day, you can start taking it kinda easy, chilling a little. Your long run on the weekend before should be shorter and easier than your long runs leading up to this week. Take a rest day on Monday, and another one on the day before the race—usually Friday or Saturday, right? On the other days, make your workouts shorter than normal. Focus on technique. In the pool, concentrate on making your strokes long and efficient, and practice swimming a few yards at a time with your head out of the water to imitate what you'll be doing when sighting for buoys on the swim course. On the bike, work on a quick pedaling cadence and on moving the pedals round in circles. When you run, count those steps. Aim for ninety or more right foot strikes per minute, and keep your head up, your shoulders relaxed, your breathing even.

Here's a thing to think about—just because you're not a highly trained, whippet-thin elite competitor, that doesn't mean you can't practice your technique in earnest. You have just as much right to work on your skills as an Ironman champion does.

This time of easing up on your strenuous efforts and focusing mentally on the race is what the coaches call a taper. The idea is that you've worked your body hard enough—now it's time to recharge your batteries, get rested, get fresh. Your body doesn't fully realize the gains of any given workout until about ten days later, because it takes that amount of time to rebuild your muscles and supply them with extra little capillaries and such. The upshot is that any training session you do the week of the race is not going to increase your fundamental fitness in time for the big day. So if you feel all panicked and stressed that you didn't train enough, please resist the temptation to go out and ride up Devil's Six-Mile Grade in the week before the race. It'll just wear you out, and your race will suffer, and you'll have less fun. The longer your race is, the longer you taper. Ironman distance events might call for a three- or four-week taper. Also, as you get older, you may need to taper longer. Even though your first race should be a sprint distance, it's a good idea to get in the habit of gearing down your workouts for a pre-race week. It makes you feel like a steely-eyed, granite-muscled real triathlete when you can announce to your family and friends, "Oh, I only swam a mile this morning. I'm in my pre-race taper, you see."

If you have a chance, scout the course in the week or weeks preceding the race. Especially for your first race, it's worth driving a little on the weekend prior to race day so that you can get a real good look at where you're going to be and start picturing yourself in that setting. You can take note of any little twists like a sharp turn on the bike or a little uphill on the run and prepare mentally for how you'll address them on the day.

IT'S ALL IN YOUR MIND

THERE'S BEEN A lot of research done on the psychology of successful athletes. Surprisingly, we SFTs can do a lot of the same mental preparation that a Lance Armstrong or Michael Jordan does, and it can actually help our performance. Maybe we're not going to win five Tours de France (Tour de Frances?) or NBA titles, but I'm a living breathing witness to the fact that even Jayne Schmo can use her mind to have a better race. Even more importantly, it can help us have more fun while we're training and racing, so that's gotta be good, yeah? My coach, Lisa, started teaching her little flock of tri chicks about the mental side of racing pretty early in my second season. From my first race, I had always had an eager, happy approach to any race day, a sense of freedom and celebration, and a big goofy grin from the moment I got to the race site. Those are good attributes to cultivate, at least in my view. What Lisa worked on was very specific visualization and affirmation techniques.

Visualization is no more complicated than running a movie of your race through your head, looking out at the race through your eyes, going through each segment in such detail that it takes as much time to visualize the race as it does to actually do the race. When your races get a little longer, like three hours or more, you're allowed to skip over some of the middle bits and focus on key areas of the race. Start at the starting line, in your wetsuit, waiting for the starter's signal. In your mind, swim out to the first buoy. Imagine where you are in your wave. Are you going to stay at the back to avoid the crowds, or are you flinging yourself into a scrum of bodies with an inner howl of reckless abandon? I like the scrum, myself, but I'm kind of in the minority on that. Picture yourself making any turns, sighting for the next buoy and coming into the swim finish.

Especially spend some time visualizing your transitions. Hopefully you took to heart my modest pleadings in the last chapter and practiced your transitions. Now picture yourself running (or at least shuffling) into your transition area, peeling off your wetsuit and swim cap, putting on your bike shoes and helmet, and heading for the bike exit.

Visualize your bike ride, seeing yourself as natural, strong, fast, confident—whatever you like as long as it's positive. Visualizing yourself floundering in the water or puffing like a walrus on the bike is not what this exercise is about. Picture yourself pedaling smoothly, running with a balanced motion and consistent pace. Picture yourself enjoying the race. And remember, your eyes are the camera in this movie. You're not watching yourself do the race from an outside point of view, you're watching the race from your perspective as you're racing. You see the bikes in front of you, you hear the roar of the crowd to either side, you watch the finish line draw closer as you pick up your pace in exhilaration, or at least in the hope that the spectators won't realize how tired you really are.

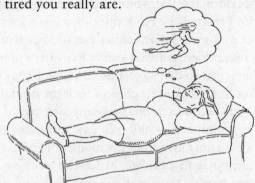

It's better to focus on what you're doing and how you feel while you're doing it than on specific time goals or passing Janelle or Bob from your club. You don't necessarily have control over those matters. The only thing that you do have control over is having the best race you can, given your ability and training. And your best race doesn't mean you smash your personal best time or place in the top ten in your age group, or even that you finish. Your best race means you gave it what you had to give on that day and you dealt with stuff as it came up.

You should also make yourself some affirmations. Now, I will be the first to raise my hand and say I always thought that crap was bogus. You know, you look in the mirror and say, "I deserve to be rich and beautiful" a hundred times, so it will come true. Yeah, right. And monkeys will fly out of my butt. That's the kind of stuff that gives us Californians a bad name. I was very skeptical indeed when Lisa assigned us the task of creating affirmations for our second race of the season. She swore that you could make up these affirmations and repeat them to yourself, or even out loud, and—here's the kicker—even if you did *not* believe them, they would sink into the nooks and crannies of your brain and propel you to greater performances in spite of your lack of faith. I said, "OK, as long as I don't have to believe them, I guess I'll try."

Lisa says that your affirmations should start with "I." That's right, this time it is all about you. So for example, "I'm strong and fast," or "I love racing," or "I feel strong in the water." Figure out what you're most worried about for your upcoming race. Is it the swim? The run? Getting your wetsuit off? Then create some affirmations that address that. "I cut through the water like a knife." "I have springs in my shoes." "My body slides out of the wetsuit like a greased pig." That sort of thing. Choose your own metaphors, of course. Or you can borrow

Lisa's generic affirmation, which has a nice rhythm to it for running: "I am awesome. I kick ass. I stay focused on my task." It's pithy and to the point.

So I repeated my affirmations to myself for a couple of days, and I chanted them out loud in the car all the way down to the race site, banging out a percussive accompaniment on the dashboard. This is probably one reason why my husband doesn't accompany me to races much. That and the 4:30 A.M. wake-up calls. And darned if I didn't have my best run ever, breaking the magical ten-minute mile barrier that I had never ever broken before. I was instantly converted. The next race I did the same thing. I ran even faster, and it felt even easier. It was weird. So give it a shot—it can't hurt. And you don't even have to believe that you're strong and fast.

IT WOULDN'T HURT TO HAVE A PLAN

IT'S ALL VERY well visualizing and affirming, being all positive and warm and fuzzy and that, but what are you actually going to *do* on race day? This is where the cold, hard, analytical side of your brain can help you out. Write up a race plan that goes from the day before the race to the time you're done. I saw this in a magazine one time and it really helps me keep my thoughts together as the big day approaches and I get all hyper.

I draw up a table that lets me put down a few notes about the physical, mental, and nutritional aspects of everything from pre-race, through the swim, T1, bike, T2, run, and post-race euphoria. Oh, here, why don't I just show you what one of mine looks like.

San Jose International Triathlon 2003 Race Plan

When	Physical/Technique	Mental	Nutrition
Saturday	20-minute easy run—quick feet. Stay off feet. Stay out of sun.	Visualize peak performance in the race. Pack car night before. Go to bed by 10 P.M.	Hydrate, hydrate, hydrate.
ACTUAL:			
Sunday A.M.		Get up 5:30 A.M. Remember to smile. Leave for San Jose 6 A.M., park at Water District.	Breakfast around 5:45 A.M.: whole grain cereal, milk.
ACTUAL:			
Pre-race 6:30–7:40 A.M.	Stay warm. Sunscreen even if cloudy. Avoid aimless wandering around. Lube up good for fast wetsuit exit. Sit still, stretch.	Set up area—gels in pocket. Thank volunteers. Scope out T1, T2 route, rack position. Scout swim course. Smile! Affirmation: "I am faster 'cause I'm fitter and I'm lighter."	Clif Bar or gel at 7:15 A.M. or when hungry. Keep drinking.
ACTUAL:			
Swim	Long, strong, smooth strokes. Push it—this is a short swim! Minimal kick. Goal: 26 minutes or better for 1,250 meters	Relaxed sighting—stay tight to buoys. Relaxed breathing. Don't be afraid to go fast here even if I feel tired. Affirmation: "I'm a swift seal in the water"	
ACTUAL:			
T1	Ruthless wetsuit exit. Run hard right out of the water. Goal: 2 minutes and 45 seconds.	Saddle carry. Make sure bike is geared down. Prepare to go fast.	
ACTUAL:			

Bike	Sit back on Bailey Hill. Get aero on flats. Aggressive on flats, downhills. Cadence up. Goal: 1:18:00 or better.	Feel strong and fast. Smile! Thank the volunteers. Enjoy the beauty of the course. Affirmation: "I can spin up Bailey and hammer everywhere else."	Drink 1 bottle Cytomax. 2 gels if possible.
ACTUAL:			
T2	Goal: 2 minutes or less.	Thank the volunteers.	Grab a gel—really! You'll want it later.
ACTUAL:			
Run	Keep cadence up. Forward lean. Relaxed upper body. Head up. Goal: 61 minutes or better.	Smile! Remember I can do sub-10s—I did it for 5 miles at UVAS. Thank the volunteers. Repeat mantras of technique, count cadence twice. Be willing to accept discomfort and keep going hard. Affirmations: "I float along the road. I am ready to set a PR [personal record] in the 10K."	Sip at aid stations-don't get bloated. Eat a gel at the halfway point, follow with water.
ACTUAL:			
Post race	Keep moving around. Stretch—really, stretch this time! Overall Time Goal: 2:49:45	Thank the volunteers. Bask in accomplishment.	Eat bananas, drink water. Drink Endurox. Eat sensibly the rest of the day.
ACTUAL:			

As you can see, I have these sort of cryptic notes to myself about what I want to do, like "Get aero on flats." That's my reminder to myself to tuck down low over my handlebars during the flat stretches of the race. "Ruthless wetsuit exit" is shorthand for, "For god's sake don't be a wimp—pull the dang thing off as hard as you can!" It actually seemed to work for that race, too. And I have to remind myself to eat sensibly the rest of the day, otherwise I look at racing as license to consume food with extreme prejudice.

The mental part of training and racing is at least as important as the physical side, if not more. And if you don't think I've made this point already, then I'm not doing a very good job writing this book and I should return my advance to the publisher. Uh-huh. But seriously, let me repeat: *Success is all in your mind.* If you intend to have a great time, and you focus on having a great time, then you're going to be a big success. Your race plan is a great place to focus on the mental aspect. I've got my overall affirmations and my bike affirmations in here, and I remind myself everywhere to smile, to have fun, to thank the volunteers who got up before dawn on a Sunday morning so that I could have water and course directions, and to enjoy the scenery around me. I figure if I can do all those things, then my race is a success no matter what my time is.

You also see that I remind myself to eat and drink specific amounts at specific times. This becomes more important the longer your race is. And in the excitement of racing, you can easily forget to eat and drink. If you're out there longer than ninety minutes, not drinking and eating can really become a problem. I'll go into that a little more in a minute.

I have time goals for all the parts of the race. This was my eighth race and I actually had a pretty good idea of what I could do and what I wanted to do timewise. I wouldn't worry about setting time goals at all if it's not important to you, or if you're just starting out and have no idea what it's going to be like. Don't stress over time if it's not fun for you. For me, it is fun. Checking my times on my watch and comparing them to my goals is a big part of the game; it keeps me entertained out there.

Finally, you'll see that I have lines marked "Actual" for every segment of the plan. After the race I go back and fill these out. It's a great way to learn about how you raced, how you felt, and what you want to do for next time. If there is a next time. I'm really hoping there will be for you and anyone else who does their first tri. This is what my planned and actual looked like for the bike and T2 of the San Jose International.

Bike	Sit back on Bailey Hill. Get aero on flats. Aggressive on flats, downhills. Cadence up. Goal: 1:18:00 or better.	Feel strong and fast. Smile! Thank the volunteers. Enjoy the beauty of the course. Affirmation: "I can spin up Bailey and hammer everywhere else."	Drink 1 bottle Cytomax. 2 gels if possible.
ACTUAL:	Got as aero as I could the whole way—headwinds made this imperative. Rode aggressively—caught great legal draft on Santa Teresa. Cadence good. Quads, hamstrings didn't cramp this time. Bailey felt pretty easy, relatively! Actual: 1:20:01– OK considering winds	Felt strong but not fast in the first half, against the wind. Smiled as soon as I turned around. The course was gorgeous! I did spin up Bailey and hammer everywhere else. I think I could have gone even a little harder on the way back in. I was trying to conserve my legs for the run.	Had a gel right at the beginning, another gel at top of Bailey. Most of bottle of Cytomax, most of small bottle of water.
T2	Goal: 2 minutes or less.	Thank the volunteers.	Grab a gel—really! You'll want it later.
ACTUAL:	Actual: 1 minute and 41 seconds, *Yay!* I took my feet out of shoes before T2 and ran like crazy in socks. Could have been faster if I had run the right way out of bike rack. D'oh!	Can't remember if I thanked them or not. Definitely having fun in this T2.	Had a gel in my pocket.

Looking back at this table, it really brings the whole race back to me. I remember dreading Bailey Hill, making my affirmation to ward against my fear, and how it didn't seem so bad on the day. And I remember the guy I tailed for miles, sitting the legal two bike lengths between his back wheel and my front wheel. Thanks, dude, you were a big help.

So that's fun. Tick, tick, tick, the clock is marking off the hours and the minutes before the horn goes off.

THREE DAYS BEFORE

LADIES AND GENTLEMEN, start loading carbos! Unfortunately for the more gluttonous of us, this is not a license to go out and scarf as much pasta as you can swallow for three days. And if you project that your race time is going to be less than ninety minutes total, don't even bother with the carbo-load.

The idea behind carbo-loading is that your body uses a sugar called glycogen for fuel. There's enough of it stored in your muscles and liver to keep you going for about ninety minutes. If you go out longer than an hour and a half without topping up the sugars, you'll bonk. What is bonking, you ask? Webster's defines it as "to strike" or "to cause to come into contact with," whereas in the UK it's slang for "to have sexual intercourse with." Endurance athletes know bonking as "hitting the wall." You get tired, shaky, weak, and generally unable to continue exerting yourself.

Eating plenty of carbohydrates in the few days before a race helps ensure that you have a full load of glycogen on board so that you can postpone the bonk as long as possible. The nutrition gurus would beg you to take in your carbs in the form of whole grains and fruits, rather than in the form of cookies and potato chips. Also, eat some lean protein and plenty of veggies. Your body needs these things.

If your race plan isn't done yet, better get a start on that.

TWO DAYS BEFORE

GET A GOOD night's sleep tonight 'cause you may have a hard time sleeping the night before your race. You'll either feel like a kid who can't wait for Christmas morning, or like a kid who's looking forward to a dentist appointment. Either way it's tough to get your beauty rest. Try and get as much of your puttering-around-the-house and race-prep stuff done as you can so you don't spend the whole day before your race going, "Oh, dude, where are my spare inner tubes?" and "Oh, crap, I have to do my laundry."

Go over your race checklist (see sidebar—and did anyone really think I could write a triathlon book and not include a race checklist? It cannot be done. It is humanly impossible). Start putting things together in a pile, and figure out what you have to go buy at the store. Sunscreen? Inner tubes? A pump? A bike? A clue? A life?

This might be the day where you do just a short, easy run or bike ride, enough to get your legs moving and warm you up, but not enough to make you fatigued.

THE DAY BEFORE

STAY CALM. STAY off your feet. Do some stretching. Pack your race bag. Practice deep, slow breathing and visualize yourself having a great time and a good race. Repeat your affirmations. Go into the bathroom and say them out loud to the mirror.

You probably have to drive to the race site or to a park or somewhere on this day to pick up your race packet. Some races will mail out packets, but most make you pick them up the day before. Your packet should have a number for your bike, a number for your body, and possibly number stickers for your bike helmet. It may also have a cool little timing chip with a Velcro strap that attaches to your ankle. The chip beeps and records your time when you cross over wired mats at the starts and finishes of each leg of the race. Do not lose your chip! If packet pick-up is at the race site, check out where the transition area is going to be and where you might park in the morning. Also, find out when your wave is going to start. Usually the elite racers—those with a legitimate shot at winning the race—go off first, and then the rest of the swimmers go off in waves, usually based on age and gender, about five to ten minutes apart. Your race packet should have a swim cap, and the color of your cap usually determines your wave.

You may also have other goodies in the race packet—free energy bars, coupons for local eateries, and your race T-shirt. I have a superstition that I don't wear the race T-shirt until I've done the race. I made an exception once when it was freezing on race morning, and the T-shirt was the only extra layer I could put on. Nothing bad happened. Sometimes you might get a water bottle or a hat. There's this triathlete dentist in my area who donates toothbrushes to race packets. We may be slow and/or fat, but by golly our teeth are immaculate. And there will be ads, lots of ads, in your bag. Do with them what you will.

Discard the fluff. Get ready to number your bike. You can attach the number to the bike wherever you want, as long as it's readable and not in the way of important things like your pedals. The race packet usually includes extra-long twist ties for the number. I usually end up punching an extra hole in the number so I can tie it on the way I want it. This is legal.

If you have helmet stickers, stick them on the front and back of your helmet. This helps the photographers identify you and you can get your post-race photos back more easily. Your number for the run can either get safety-pinned to your top or shorts, or you can attach it to a race belt. I think I've made my feelings about safety pins perfectly clear.

Get the race information from your race packet or the race Web site and make sure you have the directions clear. Nothing sucks like getting lost on race morning. Your carefully cultivated veneer of calm will go directly to hell, and, more importantly, you run the risk of not passing go and not collecting your finisher's medal, if you get lost badly enough. If you're confused, call the race director.

Pack the bag that will go with you into the transition area. Bear in mind that you have a limited amount of space at the bike rack, so no giant rolling suitcases. I use a backpack so that if I have to park a ways away from the race site, I can ride my bike to the site and feel all self-contained. Stick everything you can in the car today so you don't forget it in the morning. While you're thinking about the car, make sure you have enough gas to get to the race, OK?

Lay out the clothes you're going to wear to the race site so you can find them in the morning. I usually put on my tri shorts, sports bra, tri top, socks, and running shoes and top off with some sweats or fleece against the chill, damp morning air. Of course, I live in Northern California. You may not have chill morning air in the summer. Set your alarm so that you have plenty of time to get dressed and fed and get to the race site at least an hour and a half before the race. For your very first race, I'd actually get there two hours beforehand. It gives you time to check everything out in a relaxed fashion and avoid energy-wasting headless chicken imitations.

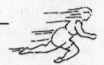

Race Day Checklist

RACE BAG:
- towel to put your stuff on
- timing chip
- race packet with instructions

SWIM:
- cap—usually provided for you by the race organizers
- goggles—stick a spare pair in, too, in case your band breaks at the last minute
- wetsuit, if you're gonna wear one
- whatever you're swimming in

BIKE:
- helmet
- bike shoes if you wear them
- sunglasses
- gloves
- water bottle with sports drink
- whatever you wear on the bike

RUN:
- shoes
- socks if you use them
- race number—on a belt or on your shirt
- hat (optional)
- whatever you wear on the run

OTHER REALLY GOOD STUFF:
- watch—oh, and make sure it's waterproof, yeah?
- sunscreen
- Bodyglide or other lube
- energy bar
- energy gel
- extra water
- ID, money
- cell phone
- camera

NOT IN YOUR RACE BAG, BUT WITH YOU:
- bike—I'm serious, I live in fear of setting off without it
- spare inner tubes in your bike bag
- clothes and shoes for after the race
- a big plastic bag for your wetsuit
- extra towel
- pumps—frame pump and floor pump
- maps, directions

So your bag's packed, your numbers are in place, you know where you're going. Kick back, enjoy, go to bed early, and we'll see you tomorrow morning.

RACE MORNING

WERE YOU ABLE to sleep? Don't worry about it. It's too late now. Once race day arrives, don't worry about anything. If there's something going on that you can control, handle it, and if you can't control it, let go completely. Come to think of it, this is pretty decent advice for all aspects of life. Some people, like my Mom, aren't happy unless they're worrying about something, but you lose a lot of energy doing this before a triathlon.

So race day arrives, you wake up in the pitch dark even in the height of summer, you stumble around with a flashlight, trying to find the clothes you laid out last night, trying not to stub your toe on the bed frame and wake your spouse with a blood-curdling howl. I hardly ever get up in the dark. It's against my religion, so race days are kind of special for me in this way.

Make sure you get up early enough so that you can eat breakfast, something with some protein and some quality carbs. Oatmeal or cereal and milk, or yogurt and a banana, or whatever you would normally eat a couple of hours before a longer workout. Today is not the day for the half-dozen Krispy Kremes or the breakfast burrito special with extra jalapeños from Juan's. Keep it wholesome and bland like your local news anchor. Fill up a water bottle and keep drinking from it.

Get your bike on or in the car, grab your race bag and water bottle, head 'em up, roll 'em out, get going. The feeling of speeding down the freeway with a car full of gear, knowing my only responsibility for the day is going to the race and having a great time, that's a major buzz for me. I get a little smile going just thinking about it. So turn up your CD player and sing a little, or repeat your affirmations as loudly and firmly as you can. This is not the time to be embarrassed. No one can hear you. Unless of course you have someone in the car with you. Then it would be a really good time to be embarrassed. Repeat affirmations to yourself, silently, if you are accompanied.

Once you get parked, top up the pressure in your bike tires so you can leave your floor pump in the car. Arrange yourself so you can ride to the race site if it's a long walk, and glide quietly through the early morning half-light with all the other silent pre-dawn figures. At the transition, find your numbered spot if there are assigned spaces, or pick out a good rack spot, preferably one as close as possible to both the bike entrance and the run exit. Lay out your towel and your transition set-up just like you practiced. Look around, take in the sights and sounds and colors and the cool air, take a deep breath, and smile broadly. This is gonna be awesome. Put your sunscreen on, even if it's cloudy. You know the UV drill.

At most races, you'll get your race number written on your arm and thigh, and your age on your calf. This is yet another advantage of having some extra flesh—it gives the body-marking volunteers more room to write the number. The volunteers will be somewhere around the transition area waiting for you to drop your sweats so they can write on you. I usually giggle like the Pillsbury Doughboy when they do, because it tickles. It sort of detracts from any type of a grim race face, if you're trying to maintain one. For me, my preferred race face is that of an excited Labrador retriever, so I'm not worrying too much about displaying ferocity or determination or anything intimidating.

So get your bod marked up, and then go check out the course. You want to figure out where you go into the water, where you come out of the water, what your route is to the transition area, and where your bike is going to be, relative to where you come in. Count the number of racks or look for a landmark to help you find your bike. Then figure out where you'll come back in on the bike, how to find your transition spot when you're coming back, and where you go to get out of transition and onto the run. Usually these spots will be marked with "Bike In" and "Run Exit" and other helpful banners.

At some point you want to maybe head over for the Porta-John. Make sure you leave enough time for the line. Keep smiling.

Once you've taken care of business, it's time to get down to fun. I usually start getting my wetsuit on at least a half hour before my wave start. This process does double duty as my warm-up, as I work up a pretty good sweat battling with the Neoprene devil. Some people like to jog around to warm up, and that's a pretty good idea. Just make sure you're not sweaty when you go to put the wetsuit on, 'cause then you will be in a pickle. For some reason it's even harder to put a dry wetsuit on a wet body than it is to put it on a dry body. The Neoprene wants to stick to your sweat or something. I haven't examined the option of getting both myself and the wetsuit wet before trying to put it on. If you haven't been practicing putting the suit on, shame on you, but allow an extra few minutes just in case. Depending on your body type, your wet-suit might just slip right on. But if you're reading a book called *Slow Fat Triathlete*, and you are, it's possible that the wetsuit designers were thinking of some other body type than yours and mine when they cut the Neoprene. So lube up and be patient. Pull each leg on slowly, like a recalcitrant pair of stockings. If you've never known the joys of stockings, check with an understanding female friend—maybe she can give you a lesson.

Head over to the swim start with at least fifteen minutes to go before your wave. Check out the swim course—figure out where the buoys are and what side you have to pass them on. Watch a couple of waves go off and see how they swim. Jump in the water and splash around, make some noise, swim a few strokes to get your groove on. This is where my usual warm-up takes place. Also, the cold water will make you want to pee in your wetsuit. To coin a phrase: Just do it. You've been hydrating for days, your pee is almost clear, and the water will wash it all out anyway. Now is not the time for niceties of etiquette.

Keep an eye on the other swimmers with your color swim cap on, and an eye on your watch. When your wave gets in the water, you want to be with it. Position yourself wherever you feel most comfortable. For a lot of first-timers, and even fifteenth-timers, the mellowest place to be is at the back of the wave, away from the flailing arms and legs. If you're a strong swimmer or have a background in rugby or wrestling, get right on up there in front and put your nose in.

Listen for the starter. You'll probably be standing in the water or on the beach. Look around. Have another big smile. Repeat your swim affirmation to yourself. Breathe deeply. If this is your first triathlon, you'll remember it forever. The starter will count you down, and you'll be racing! Finally, in the middle of the fifth chapter! Oh, yeah, and as you move forward into your swim, hit the "start" button on your watch's stopwatch function.

As the swim starts, you'll notice that the water has been transformed into a vat full of giant black squid, all waving their tentacles at you and trying to stop you from moving forward. Relax, find yourself a patch of water, and just start swimming. You may get jostled, grabbed, bumped, or kicked, but try not to let it freak you out. Keep on swimming. It'll thin out soon enough. Go out at a relaxed pace. You don't want to blow all your energy in the first two minutes of the race. You can always pick it up in a little while once you're used to the fact that you're racing. Now lift your head up and check for your first buoy. Don't keep your head up there forever, just long enough to catch a glimpse of it. Swim, kick a little, relax, breathe. Sight again. Just keep doing that until you get near the end of the course.

As you approach the land, start thinking about your transition: how you're going to reach for your wetsuit zipper, what direction you're going to run in once you get out of the water. Swim until your hand touches bottom, then, just before you get up, grab the neck of your wetsuit and tug it open a little, letting some water in. This will loosen up the suit and make it easier to shuck off. Stand up, wobble out of the water, and head for your bike. Remember, you'll be dizzy, but don't worry, it will pass. The most common triathlon technique is to get the upper half of the wetsuit off while you're jogging to the bike, but there's no law. You can sit down as soon as you get out of the water and work your suit off. Or you can run to your bike and then take the whole thing off. Or you can swim without a wetsuit and avoid all these difficult decisions.

Try and dump the wetsuit somewhere where it won't get trampled on too much, get your helmet on, get your shoes on, and head out. Remember to take your swim cap and goggles off before you leave. Now you're on your way. This is fun, huh? Remember, you usually have to run with your bike until the volunteers tell you it's safe to get on. And now it's just like riding a bike. Keep your gearing low and your legs moving at a fast cadence. Get them warmed up. Watch your position on the road and relative to other cyclists, and watch out for the good people directing traffic.

The bike course is the bit where the rules of triathlon really matter. Here are the key ones:

- Ride on the right, pass to the left. Never pass to the right of another rider. It's a penalty and it can get you disqualified.
- Ride as far to the right as is practicable. If there's room on the right for people to pass you, then you're too far to the left—get over.
- Never, ever, ever cross the center line of a road into oncoming traffic. You'll get disqualified, and you could be killed.
- Avoid drafting—getting too close to the person in front of you, which allows you to cut the wind resistance you face by a dramatic amount. It's a key technique in bike racing, but it's considered cheating in age-group triathlon competition. The front of your front wheel has to be at least two bike lengths behind the end of the back wheel in front of you. If someone passes you, it's your responsibility to drop back to a legal position.

▶ Don't throw anything on the course except near an aid station. You can get a penalty, and what's worse, you'll be littering.

Be cool, be smart, and listen to the volunteers, and you'll have a great time.

Pedal, breathe, drink some sports drink, maybe eat an energy gel about forty minutes into your race. Look around a little and enjoy the scenery. Thank the volunteers as they hand you water or Gatorade. Before you know it, you'll be almost back at transition. As you approach, think about where your bike rack is and where you're going to run to. Maybe stand up on the pedals, stretch your legs out a little. Start thinking of yourself as a runner.

Slow down and get off the bike as the volunteers direct you. Head over to your spot, hang up your bike, and whip off your helmet and shoes. Slip into your running shoes, grab your race number and hat, and go. Don't be like me—make sure you run in the right direction out of the bike rack. It's OK that your legs feel like new and improved lead flavor Jell-O, you'll remember that from your brick workouts. Just keep shuffling forward, and that feeling will go away eventually.

Check this out, boo! You're almost done with your first race! Just a little jog through the park and you're home free. Keep your head up and your feet moving. Do a little exercise where you count your right foot steps for a minute. If you're below ninety, work on moving your feet a little faster. You don't have to take bigger steps; in fact, you should take smaller steps and concentrate on leaving your feet on the ground for the shortest possible time. I know you've been working on this throughout your training. This is just a reminder.

Most races have aid stations with water and maybe Gatorade set up every mile or so. Take a little of one or the other, or both. My advice is to walk while you drink. If I concentrate very hard, I can jog and drink at the same time, but it tends to make me feel weird and bloated in the belly region. Walk a few steps, drink, then keep it going. Repeat every mile.

After the first mile or so, you should have your regular legs back after the bike ride's rubberizing effects wear off. My only advice now is to keep moving, keep smiling, keep thanking the volunteers, and keep remembering to look around you and take in the spectacle. You're doing something you may have thought you could never do.

If your chest is heaving and your legs are burning, that's just about right. Keep doing that. If you can't keep that up, back off for a bit. You still have to make it all the way to the end. Take a walk break if you have to, but keep pushing forward.

After an amount of time that will seem incomprehensibly long, you will see the finish line. Make sure your race number's hanging cleanly in the front, pick your head up, and look like you're having fun because someone will certainly be taking your picture. It's pretty normal to put on a final finishing spurt when you smell the barn, but take care not to pull any muscles in your excitement.

No matter how tired you are, muster up a huge grin as you step over that line. You did it. You're a finisher, a triathlete, a superhero. You need to be really, really proud of yourself.

POST-RACE

AND NOW, QUICKLY, you need to drink a bunch of water and get some calories into you. Keep moving around, head for the refreshment area, and scoop up as much as you can carry of whatever seems good to you. Bagels, bananas, oranges, and sports drinks are pretty common post-race fare, and they'll help your muscles to recover faster. Seriously. Start eating right away. Don't go totally ape, but definitely eat the equivalent of a bagel or thereabouts. Thank the volunteers who got up on Sunday morning to serve you food.

Once you've eaten, take a few minutes to stretch a little. Be very, very gentle. All your muscles are exhausted and you could hurt yourself if you stretch too quickly or vigorously. But if you don't stretch at all, you'll feel like the Tin Woodman tomorrow, and there won't be any oil around.

Also, you need to be alert for the inevitable onset of Post-Race Stupidity Syndrome (PRSS). Problem is, it will happen to you, and then you won't be alert. PRSS, though widespread, is usually not too serious and is almost always temporary, though I am beginning to believe in a Post-Post-Race Stupidity Syndrome Syndrome, which is cumulative in its effects. The symptoms of PRSS include not being able to find your bike after the race, and then, when you do eventually find it, you stand staring at your scattered, wet gear without the slightest idea of how to pack it back into your suddenly tiny race bag. You may also forget where you put your car keys, where you live, what your name is, or other details. It's not an unpleasant sensation, but just keep in mind that the rest of the day may not be a good time to discuss finances with your spouse or do anything that requires analytical ability, decisiveness, or anything other than good-natured apathy. Just smile wanly and say, "I'm so sorry honey, but I have acute PRSS at the moment. Can we postpone this discussion for a day or so?"

Experts disagree on the exact cause of PRSS. OK, they don't, really, 'cause I made it up, but every triathlete I've talked to agrees that it exists. We hypothesize that it's a combination of physical exhaustion, the after-effects of having your body flooded with adrenaline from the time you woke up in the very early morning, the relief of having finished the race, and the dissolution of the intense mental focus you've been maintaining at least all day, and maybe for the last couple of days. I mean, look at all the stuff I told you to do and think about and remember just for this little sprint race today. No wonder your brain is toast. Just relax and enjoy it. There is no cure but time, a soft couch, and a lot of sports on TV. Actually, I'm told the sports on TV part is optional, but it's not for me.

One thing that will help heal your body, though it will make your mushy brain feel even mushier, is to soak in a hot bath with about three cups of Epsom salts dissolved in the water. It's a pretty miraculous way to help stave off muscle soreness. I know this because I did my first six or seven races without it. When I did get the tip, I couldn't believe how much better I felt after that Epsom salts bath.

When your PRSS has abated, take a little while to reflect on your accomplishment. How do you feel now that you've done the race? What have you learned about yourself? Are you more disciplined than you thought you were? Do you have a bulldog streak of competitiveness that you didn't know about? Are you a screaming wimp about cold water? Go back to your race plan and fill in the "Actual" rows. What was the race like compared to your expectations and your carefully laid plans?

You might even want to take to the computer or the journal and write up a little race report. Share with your family and friends, let them know what this day was like for you. What were you afraid of? Did it happen? What was the most amazing moment? What was the funniest thing that happened? They will probably be amazed and awed, and you'll feel like the hero of your own story, which you are.

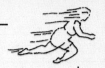

The Slow Fat Triathlete
Recommends

Again, I'm just repeating the points I feel like I didn't hammer on enough earlier in the chapter.

1. Don't change it. Whatever it is, in the couple of weeks before a race, don't change it unless it's a flat tire or a thrashed pair of socks. Don't test out new bike gear or new shoes or a new sports drink the day of a race, or even the week of a race.

2. Use your mind, grasshopper. Spend time before the race visualizing yourself having fun and feeling good during the race. Make up some affirmations and repeat them constantly. "I am fast enough." "I feel good about my preparation." "I am Godzilla, storming through the water, trampling the land." Whatever works for you.

3. Make a list, check it twice. You really want to feel confident that you have everything you need, including directions to the race site.

4. Sleep well two nights before the race. The night before, you may not be able to sleep so well, but it doesn't matter.

5. Make having fun and staying injury free your ultimate race day goals.

6. Recover fully. This includes eating and drinking right after you finish your race so that you get rehydrated and replenished with glycogen, moving around, stretching, taking an Epsom salts bath the night after the race, and staying away from hard training until you feel "normal" again.

6

GOING THE EXTRA MILE OR 124.5

OPTIONS FOR CONTINUING YOUR
ATHLETIC ENDEAVORS

THAT WAS AMAZING, dude! You did your race and you had a blast. You're a triathlete. You rock! In your euphoria and exhaustion you're lighter than a helium balloon and heavy as a sandbag. You're sweating and sunburned and covered in algae and salt. Frankly, you're disgusting. But you don't care, and neither do I. You should take a good long time to bask in your accomplishment. I remind myself to do this by writing "Bask in my accomplishment" in the post-race section of every race plan. This usually manifests itself in hugging everyone I know or think I maybe know or think I might like to get to know (just kidding, Tim). There's also a lot of grinning and dancing to whatever music the race directors might be playing. I sing and play drums on my steering wheel as I drive home from the race.

You did your race. You basked in your accomplishment. You should probably take a couple of days off training, depending on how sore you are the next day. I find the Jacuzzi at the Y even more attractive than usual the day after a race. I try and wear comfortable clothes as much as possible, and I sleep even more than I normally do for a couple of days. Racing at maximum effort is pretty stressful on your body. As the week progresses, you will start to come around. Your PRSS will wear off, although I feel that each race leaves a little divot in my brain for a while.

And now you will start to evaluate whether you have gotten the bug. If your first thought after getting your water and banana at the finish line was, "Dang, that was cool! When can I do another one?" that would be a warning sign. Thinking, "Man, next time I know I can do better on the swim" is another symptom. When the bug bites, I don't know what the cure is. You just have to let the malady run its course. Warn your loved ones that they are in for the long haul. You may develop erratic behavior, getting up before dawn to squeeze in workouts and squandering perfectly good Saturday mornings on longer and longer bike rides, returning limp-haired and liberally smeared with bicycle grease. You have no choice in the matter.

What are the options for those so afflicted? Oh, my friends, the world is wide and full of tasty fruits for those who want to pursue the tri life. You can become a sprint distance specialist, get in and out in an hour, hour and a half, get back to your car before your latte gets cold. You can do a few more sprints and step up to the international distance. You could set your sights on a half-Ironman distance race, or contemplate the rigors of the full Ironman. For these latter two options, I would recommend you have some fun at the shorter distances first, 'cause training for and racing the long courses is another kind of fun entirely. Some people get all geeked up and go ahead and train for a half in their first season, but that's pretty extreme for a slow fat triathlete. We SFTs need to build up our bodies, get 'em used to the pounding and the demands of training.

There are also off-road triathlons, where you careen around on your mountain bike and run on trails. There are duathlons, for people who just never got happy putting their faces in the water. Duathlons consist of a run leg, a bike leg, and then another run leg. This is not for me, but a lot of people seem to like it. And then there are adventure races, exercises in sleep deprivation, navigation, and confusion for teams of people even crazier than I have yet shown myself to be. Consider this—adventure racers unwrap their energy bars and then stick them to the top tubes of their mountain bikes. They eat a bite then stick the bar back on. Can you say, "Ick"? Yeah, I know. I gotta do this some day.

SPRINT—A MISNOMER FOR SOME

THE SO-CALLED sprint distance triathlon is kind of a misnomer for me. I don't think I have ever finished one in under an hour and twenty minutes, and what kind of sprint goes on for an hour and twenty minutes, I ask you? For the slow fat triathlete, every triathlon is an endurance event. So spending some time, or your whole triathlon life, specializing in the sprint distances is an entirely honorable way to go. You can focus on getting faster, on improving your technique in the different disciplines, or just on making the whole thing less painful. There are loads of sprint distance races around, the entry fees are a little cheaper and the T-shirts are just as good, or just as ugly. Don't feel any pressure to go longer if you don't want to. You can have just as much fun, maybe more, by staying short and sweet.

In case you've forgotten the first chapter, the usual sprint distance is around a 400-yard swim, a 12- or 12.5-mile bike, and a 3.1-mile or 5-kilometer run. These distances do vary a bit, but that's the general ballpark. Sprint race enthusiasts love the fact that you can be done in an hour to an hour and a half and still get home in time to catch the ball game. Also, once you get used to that distance and get into better shape, you may find that you suffer less acutely from PRSS for the rest of the day.

SPRINT PLUS

A LOT OF times, race directors want to put on a nice little race, but the course they have in mind just doesn't fall neatly into one of the standard boxes. These guys and gals embody the original crazy-ass spirit of triathlon, so I'm going to salute them for refusing to be pigeonholed, categorized, pinned to a card like a beetle in a collector's case. So you see a number of races where the swim is 800 yards, the bike is 16 miles, and the run is 3 miles, like the Shelbyville Triathlon in Shelbyville, Indiana, or the East Canyon Triathlon in Utah, with a 1,000-meter swim, 14-mile bike, and 3-mile run. For you folks who loathe the swim but like the bike, there's this race in Vass, North Carolina, that's 300 yards in the water, 20 miles on the bike, and another 3.1 jogging through the country club.

And therein lies the beauty of the sprint plus races. They have this delightful obstreperous variety and you can pick your poison. If you spent your summers at swim camp but can't get comfortable on your bike, find a race with a swim that's proportionately longer. And also go to a good bike shop to see if they can help you get comfortable on the bike.

INTERNATIONAL DISTANCE

I WANT TO call this Olympic distance, but the International Olympic Committee and Mr. Samaranch might have to pause in their inveterate perk grubbing to hunt me down and maim me for life. You know how those Olympic folks can be, bless their hearts. So we'll review— the international distance (hey, legal department, can we say "Oly"?) or Oly distance is a 1,500-meter swim, a 40-kilometer bike ride, and a 10-kilometer run. I did three sprint distance races before attempting an Oly, and lots of people do that or more. By the way, the Olympic distance is the distance they race in the Olympics. It's just under a mile swim, about 26 miles on the bike, and then 6.2 miles of running.

This is a really popular distance in my neck of the woods. It's long enough to test your endurance, but short enough to be within the reach of a first- or second-year slow fat triathlete. Fast people (I've seen them, I see their dust rising in the distance) do these races in under two hours. My best time is around three, but four-plus is not uncommon. The nice thing about this is that you can contemplate these distances without blanching and popping your eyes out of your head. Maybe right now the idea is pretty eye-popping, but hey, once you've trained for a sprint distance, you may well feel that the Oly distance is within your reach in the not-too-distant future. In your training, you may well have done some longer distances than your sprint race required, just to feel confident that you could do them without collapsing in an unsightly heap. So if you had done a 16- or 17-mile ride, say, well, then you're practically there! That's the approach to getting longer: Just sneak up on it real quiet and easy, so the distance doesn't spook you.

If you do an international distance race, you can also justify a slightly longer drive to get there. In my first season, I had two races where I drove four and five-and-a-half hours round trip to do races that I finished in about 1:20 and 1:27 respectively. I had a blast at both races cause I always do, but think how much more fun I could have had if I'd been able to race for three hours instead. Yeah, yippee, I hear you say. Well, you know, if you don't get the bug, you're probably not even reading this chapter. Or you might race a few more sprint distances and then decide, you know, I really would like to extend the amount of time I get wet, sweaty, sunburned, chafed, blistered, and exhausted. And then you'll sign up for an Oly race and you'll have a great time.

A Sidebar About Pain

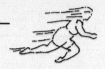

Pain is an interesting topic, in general. For one thing, there are so many different kinds of pain, and the triathlete may have the opportunity to experience several of them. Pain is probably what people fear when they face training and racing. People like me don't help, writing about burning legs and ribs that ache from the strain of breathing. Lance Armstrong is widely quoted about the purifying effects of suffering. And the pain that really burned the sport of triathlon into the consciousness of the American sports viewer was Julie Moss's collapse and crawl to the finish of Ironman Hawaii in 1982. She was in a lot of pain. If you go all out in a race situation and you really want to test yourself, you can feel pretty uncomfortable.

For the beginning triathlete, don't even go there. You don't want to work hard enough to really hurt until you've got a pretty good base of fitness. And you may never want to work that hard. But you should definitely go easy on yourself as you work up to your first races and even as you race, otherwise you risk feeling some other kinds of pain—a pop or twinge that means injury, or the lingering aches of an overuse injury. Those kinds of pain are not good. Now, again, this is a "Do as I say, not as I do" situation. The very first time I went out and did a 5K fun run, I ran the last mile so hard I feared losing my breakfast, and I still pretty much finish up that way every time I race. But that's the pain of hard effort, which is an entirely different animal.

Not that the pain of hard effort is necessarily good. But it ain't necessarily bad, either. If you have the training in, including short intervals of training at high intensity (read "pain"), you can work on going hard in your races and just kind of dealing with how it feels. It's one of those mental training things. You're coming toward the end of your race and it's getting tough. So your legs are getting tired—it's cool. It'll be over soon. So your energy is flagging and your chest is heaving. Don't fight it. Try and experience it. This is what it feels like at this level of effort. You're not going to die. (If you do die, you're going too hard.) You'll get over it when you stop. So just see how long you can keep going before you stop. Try reveling in the power of your body to keep going under stress. One Web site I read advised picturing your healing mental energy as a glowing ball of light, which you can send to your legs when they start to hurt. Whatever, dude. Another one I've heard is, "It's not pain, it's just the sensation of competing hard." And for some reason that kind of hits home for me.

As you move along your triathlon journey, take some time to think about that pain. Do you want to avoid it? Or is there some weird way in which that maximum effort is fun for you? Would you enjoy this more if it didn't hurt at all? Or would that be too much like Play Station 2?

Just some thoughts.

HALF-IRONMAN

AGAIN, THE LEGAL department has to check on my terminology. The World Triathlon Corporation has trademarked the term "Ironman," and it's gotten its attorneys all over race directors who want to call their really long races "Ironman," so you now have such euphemisms as "iron distance" and "ultra-distance triathlon." I suspect they may have gotten their sticky fingers into the half-Ironman pie as well, since a lot of races call themselves "long course" now, although many hold out and boldly proclaim that they are half-Ironman races. I'm not going to name them in case I get them in trouble. Just go to Google and type in "half-ironman." But what you really want to think about is how long this is. The swim is 1.2 miles, the bike is 56, and the run is 13.1. Oh, my.

Many, many people are dedicated triathletes and never go anywhere near this distance. They concentrate on getting faster at shorter distances, or they have physical issues that preclude the kind of pounding your body takes during this kind of event. They may just be eminently sensible folks who think that six or seven hours of sustained effort just ceases to be fun after a while. And of course I have the utmost respect for that viewpoint. Because what is it ultimately all about? That's right. Fun.

I did my first "half" in September of my second season. And that's all I've done so far. It was an incredible experience, and it was really hard, even though I'd put in ten or eleven hours of training a week for the previous seven months. There were moments when I felt like I wasn't really having fun, although the overall day was an amazing thing. It took me about a week to get over the general fatigue, just like getting over a case of the flu, although the muscle soreness wore off in a couple of days, pretty much. And about two weeks later the second toe on my right foot still felt like someone had taken a hammer and pounded it several thousand times. Oh, right, that was me. Damn, I hate it when that happens. But the glow I felt afterwards, floating in the ocean to cool off, was more than just sunburn, and it hasn't really worn off yet. You can read all about that at the end of this chapter, and maybe it will inspire you or scare you out of any notions you may have had of attempting this one day.

The half is not something you want to approach lightly. You really need to build up your endurance over time. You have to make your knees and ankles and feet resilient. You have to train your rear end to sit on a bike saddle for three hours or so. And you really need to want to. If it's all you can do now to jog half a mile, a half-Ironman is definitely at least a couple of years away for you, no matter how much you want to. But hey, what a goal to work toward. About three years ago, I set a goal of running a marathon by my fortieth birthday. Then I got sucked into this triathlon thing instead and ended up doing a half-Ironman a little after I hit the magic forty mark. It was worth the wait. I'll definitely do another one, and probably a lot more than that, but it will entail a lot of planning and training and work. That marathon will have to wait. That's 26.2 miles—doesn't that seem long? It does to me.

IRONMAN. DUDE.

OK, SO IF you've done the math or remember the first chapter, congratulations. You have figured out that the Ironman distance is 2.4 miles of swimming, 112 miles of cycling, and then you finish that up with a nice marathon, 26.2 miles. Doesn't that sound jolly? And you only have seventeen hours to do it in; otherwise you don't get an official finish. Harsh!

These races are so incredibly demanding that a lot of people who finish one get a tattoo of the Ironman logo. I don't blame them one bit. I'm sure getting the tattoo hurts a lot less than the race, and it's over a lot quicker. The world record for this distance is around eight hours. A thirteen- or fourteen-hour race is considered quite respectable.

Maybe one day you or I will do something that requires this much determination. I know otherwise normal people who've done it. I think it's in my plans for the next couple of years. I also think that the thing that took the most determination in my life was getting into shape to run three miles in thirty-five minutes or so. Once I conquered that Everest, the rest has been a matter of gradual degrees. So, you know, think about it. Give yourself some time. Maybe put yourself on a five-year plan. Remember how well that worked for Stalin's Soviet Union? You don't? Well, they got a lot of rural electrification done during those times. This year, the sprint distances. Next year, Olympic. Year after that, maybe a half, maybe two. (Sad but true—two half-Ironman races do not add up to a full Ironman.) Your fourth year, try a mix of races, hire a coach, and look at the whole year as a training campaign. Year five—find an Ironman and give it a go! Yee-haw daddy!

Actually, you should figure out which Ironman you'll aim for sometime in year four, for two reasons. One is you will be scheduling your training pretty specifically for the race. The other is that you need to enter pretty early for the more popular North American races. Ironman Canada, the second oldest Ironman in the world, pretty much sells out a year in advance. The day after each IM Canada, registration opens for next year, and it takes one day to sell out. The way to get in is to have a friend who does the race get in line for you the day afterwards and sign you up. I'm not kidding.

And if you were thinking of taking a nice jaunt to the Kona coast to do your big race at the Granddaddy of Them All in Hawaii, take a number. You can qualify by finishing high in your age group at a number of sanctioned qualifying races, or you can enter the lottery for one of a couple hundred slots. Guess which path I'm taking. Even if you do win the lottery, you have to prove that you can do at least a half Ironman to actually make it to the starting line. But definitely give it a shot.

I hear Ironman Wisconsin is nice, and Ironman Coeur d'Alene in Idaho. Ironman Lake Placid is another famous race, and Ironman Florida has the advantage of being almost completely flat. Then there are other "iron-distance" races around the country, which are also mighty fine events.

DUATHLON—NOT GOOD FOR DUCKS

DUATHLON IS A cousin of triathlon that eliminates that whole swimmy thing. You run, you get on your bike and ride, then you get off your bike and run some more. You see a lot of these races in the spring and fall when it's just too dang cold to get in the water. Duathlons are also handy to produce because you don't need any convenient body of water. A lot of people have a lot of fun doing these. For me, being a velocity-challenged runner, skipping the swim takes half the fun out of it. The other half is the bike ride, and the run's just not fun at all. Well, I'm learning to love it, but it's definitely the hardest part. You're lying down when you're swimming, for crying out loud. How hard can that be? And you're sitting down when you're riding your bicycle. But running? You are doing *all* the work. And the more weight you carry, the more work you do.

So check out those duathlons and let me know how you like 'em. That's really all I have to say.

OFF-ROAD TRIATHLONS

WHAT COULD BE more fun than doing all this swimming, biking, and running? Maybe taking the whole bike and run onto the trail, to add rocks, tree roots, mud, and poisonous plants to the list of obstacles. Off-road triathlons bring an added element of adventure, usually get you even closer to some gorgeous scenery, and give you a chance to use your carefully honed mountain biking skills. They can also be steeper and gnarlier than road tri races.

My friend Indigo described her first off-road race as "more running than anything else. You had to run between laps of the swim, run to your bike, and then run with your bike over a lot of the bike course because it was so steep, and then you had to run on the run, too." Did she like that? "It was *soooo* much fun!" My only off-road race was my first tri, and it was only partly off the road, so I really don't have a lot to add to this section. I would love to do more mountain-bike triathlons, but unfortunately I don't own a mountain bike, and I think my husband's good will might be stretched past its ample boundaries if I added yet another bicycle to the collection on the patio.

KIDS' TRIATHLONS

YOU'RE PROBABLY TOO old to compete in these, but it's a great way to get your kids into the sport so they can have some war stories to share with Mom and Dad. My tri club has put on a kids' tri for a few years now and it is more fun than a barrelful of monkeys. Actually, it is kind of a barrelful of monkeys. Our youngest competitors, some as young as four, get lifted out of the pool, come charging out onto the bike course with their tassels on the handlebars of the pink bikes, and they have no idea where they're going. It's awesome. Even if you don't have kids, it's worthwhile going to volunteer at a kids' race 'cause you'll laugh your butt off. In a nice way, of course. Race organizers will set up the courses so that the distances are appropriate to the kids' ages, and they'll also be paying extra attention to having a super-safe bike course.

ADVENTURE RACING FROM MUDDY BUDDY TO ECO-CHALLENGE

IF MERELY SWIMMING, biking, and running off-road is too tame, try adventure racing. It combines the adrenaline insanity of X-games extreme sports with the endurance insanity of triathlon. Throw in a healthy dose of navigating, sleep deprivation, and the dynamics of a stressed out team, and things get very crazed very quickly. I definitely want to get into this sport. It reminds me of doing rafting trips in Siberia, minus the vodka.

How did this crazy stuff even get started? Some nutty French folks started doing these Raids Gauloises things, which as far as I can figure were all about stealing each other's cigarettes in the wilderness, and then there was the Eco-Challenge, and then everyone was doing it.

Founded in 1989 by French journalist and adventure dude Gerard Fusil, the Raid Gauloise is an annual event where mixed teams of men and women, four or five to a team, struggle through almost a week of intensely rugged wilderness terrain. They might run, trek, climb up steep cliffs, ride camels, paddle canoes, use perilous rope bridges to cross dizzying gorges, or all of the above and many more fiendish disciplines to get to the end. To finish, the team has to arrive at the line together. Sleep deprivation, horrendous foot rot and blistering, chafed butts, bruises, sprains, and broken bones make most triathlons look super-plush in comparison. And you have to navigate your own way from checkpoint to checkpoint.

An interesting note: In 1992, Mark Burnett captained the first American team to enter the Raid Gauloise. That same Mark Burnett was inspired to create the Eco-Challenge race, which in turn begat its own hellish spawn: Survivor. So the French are ultimately responsible for the wave of ghastly reality TV shows that made the networks of the early naughts so very perilous in prime time.

But once again, I digress. The Raids and the Eco-Challenge are like the Ironman of adventure racing. They're the oldest, and the longest, and the toughest, and you have to be right at the top of the sport even to qualify for them. So what's available to the burgeoning triathlete who fancies getting a little dirtier and a little more gonzo? Oh, lots of great stuff.

One of the most popular entries to adventure sports is the Brooks Muddy Buddy series. To me this title has a slight overtone of mud-fetish porn, but it's really a different kind of good clean dirty fun. Two-person teams compete on a 10K course—that's 6.2 miles, remember? While one rides the mountain bike, the other scrambles over obstacles, sloshes through mud pits, and crawls through tunnels. Then the biker and scrambler switch roles for more of the same. The mud pit really is a huge pile of slop, leaving competitors uniformly brown and inexplicably delighted. One advantage to the Muddy Buddy, besides the mud, is that you don't have to know how to read a map. The Muddy Buddy races hit nine US cities in its second year, showing every sign of expanding further in the years to come.

A notch up from the Buddies in distance and required skills is the Balance Bar Adventure Sprints Series. These twenty-milers get a little tougher, as teams of three have to navigate the course, as well as paddle a boat and complete some "special tests." The tests have included climbing twelve-foot walls, assembling a puzzle while blindfolded, or crawling through a maze of ropes to retrieve your mountain bike. These little games are supposed to test your ingenuity and teamwork, but I have strong suspicions that they are included to make spectators laugh their asses off. Oh, yeah, they might throw some mud pits at you in these races, too. Middle of the pack teams would take six to eight hours to complete one of these bad boys, again stretching the definition of the term "sprint" way past its limits.

If you'd like to add sleep deprivation to the list of delights, see if you can hook up with a twenty-four-hour adventure race. Balance Bar has a few, then there's the Wild Onion in New York and Los Angeles, and its smaller cousin the Wild Scallion in Chicago and Indianapolis. The Balance Bar races include mountain biking, trekking, kayaking, climbing/rappelling, and navigation. So whip out your compasses, correct for the difference between magnetic north and true north, and get busy.

The adventure racing community is growing fast and furiously, and now there are a bunch of off-road entrepreneurs who offer adventure racing training camps everywhere from San Jose to Kentucky. These helpful folks will take your money, starting at about five hundred dollars and ranging up from there, and teach you how to read a topographical map, use a compass, rappel down a cliff, mountain bike in the pitch dark, and other extremely useful skills. It sounds well worth the money to me. Or you could get together with your crazy friends and figure it all out by yourselves. Part of the adventure.

GO MONOSPORT

YOU MAY DECIDE after your triathlon experience, or experiences, that you want to focus on one discipline. Lance Armstrong did this, and see how well it worked out for him? You could set a goal of running a 10K, or a half-marathon, or even going for the full 26.2-mile marathon distance. Or you could get into cycling, ride a local century (100 miles) or half-century. Who knows, maybe you'll explore the moist but pleasant world of open water swimming.

DO SOMETHING ELSE ENTIRELY

ONCE YOU'VE EXPERIENCED the surge of vitality you get from doing regular exercise and the glow of accomplishment from setting a lofty goal and following through to its achievement, who knows what else you might want to tackle in the physical arena? You might become a kayaker, or a rock climber, or a red-hot salsa dancer, or a leaping, spiking volleyball demon. You might do a multi-day bike ride for charity or hike the Appalachian Trail.

It doesn't matter what you do. Just do something. Human bodies are built to move, and when you move, you experience and strengthen parts of yourself that are deep and elemental. There's an animal joy in movement, an elation that makes you want to hang your tongue out like a happy golden retriever or bound around like a young vervet monkey. When you get your body to the place where you can feel that joy, you've done yourself and everyone around you a huge favor.

That joy is more than just a physical pleasure, too. For me, when I'm exercising, it's one of the rare times when I'm completely present in the moment. I'm not thinking about what I have to do tomorrow or worrying about my bank account or going into a semi-vegetative state in front of the 'Niners game. I'm just there, doing what I'm doing, focusing on the movements and the breathing. It's immediate, it's eternal, and, of course, it's fun.

GO BACK TO THE COUCH

WHY ON EARTH would you do this? 'Nuff said.

Like I said, I've done one half-Ironman now, and it was a big jump. Here's how it went.

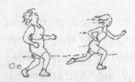

Which Half is Iron?

September 7, 2003

Big Kahuna Half-Ironman: 1.2-mile swim | 56-mile bike | 13.1-mile run
Santa Cruz, California

Once again, race morning found me up before dawn, chanting mantras of positivity and success, speeding down the highway with my bike on top of my car. I had ingested a massive bowl of oatmeal, homemade plum jam, and a banana, and I was working on a bottle of Endurox, with its highly patented ratio of carbohydrates, whey protein, and other stuff that helps you race. Basically trying to cram maximum calories down my gullet and still digest them before 7:25 A.M. And don't even think about chugging down a quarter pound of butter or something—imagine the horror that would create for your gut. It's gotta be carbos and just a little protein, pretty much no fat at all.

The reason behind this carbohydrate extravaganza was that my race was going to take just about twice as long to complete as any race I had ever done before. I estimated somewhere in the region of six and a half to seven hours and four thousand calories of energy expenditure ought to do it. Unfortunately, when you're exercising intensely, you just can't replenish the calories at nearly the rate that you burn them. If you try inhaling a burrito supreme on the bike ride, you are in for a world of hurt. Or so they say. This was my first time putting all the disciplines together into a half-Ironman distance race, and I had no idea how my digestive system was going to react to it all. I had a detailed plan involving the ingestion of sports drinks and gels and bananas at regular intervals, but it was all pretty hypothetical.

That was about to change as I bustled around, setting up my spot in the transition area, shivering a little in the wind. There was a big moment of truth coming right up, and it was going to be a six-and-a-half-hour moment. As I stood in line for the Porta-John, I tried to figure out which way the breeze was blowing and what it was going to do on the ride up to Pigeon Point and back. It appeared to be blowing straight out to sea, which seemed odd. The line for the loo was so long I didn't have time for the bike and run warm-up Coach Lisa had recommended, so I jogged around a bit and hoped for the best. I checked out the surface of the ocean and found to my delight that it was glassy as Dan Quayle's eyes. Barely a ripple.

I slithered into my wetsuit and headed over to the beach, having missed the mandatory safety meeting again. The first wave had already headed out, and I stood on the cold sand with a seasoned-looking veteran triathlete and tried to figure out the best swim route, putting off my first splash into the icy water. I did a quick "warm-up," if you can do that in sixty-two degree water, downed my last pre-race energy gel, and before I knew it the starter was counting down to "Go!"

Sometimes in a race it's the little things that make you happy. I was happy that the cold water didn't make my face hurt like it did last time I swam at Santa Cruz. And I was happy to be finally under way after all the months of training. This race was my biggest challenge of the season and I had been feeling butterflies for days. We bumped and jostled in the water—you'd think that with a whole ocean to swim in you could find three feet of clear space, but no—and I concentrated as much as I could on my stroke and my form and trying to find a similar-paced swimmer I could draft off. As usual, my drafting efforts were pretty ineffective. They say to get your hands into the bubbles from the kick of the swimmer in front of you, but once I find someone's bubbles I'm usually either on top of their feet or they're leaving me behind.

Still, I swam on and on, and things seemed to be working OK, and after a really long time I approached the beach and lurched to the upright position. The first few steps I felt wobbly, and then I hit the soft sand. Oh, Lord. I was trying to run in a barrel of taffy. This is a rude thing to do to a tired swimmer! I kept churning my legs, though, and got through the transition pretty quickly, even with having to wipe all the sand off my feet. Some races have hose wranglers to help you rinse off, or pans of water for you to run through, but I was out of luck here.

With a refreshing mixture of sand and baby powder coating the inside of my bike shoes, I tore off down Beach Street past the Coconut Grove. Amazingly, my bud Dana had not only gotten up to cheer me on at this hour on a Sunday morning, but she had convinced her friend Steph, who hardly knows me, to come, too. Wow! I passed them with a sincere thumbs-up and a big grin.

The bike course was partly familiar to me—up through the west side of town, out onto Highway One, and up and down a bunch of rollers to Davenport. But that was just the first half. The coast started to feel even more rugged as we kept heading north, and, crossing into San Mateo County, the fog and wind became palpable factors in our race. I planned on averaging at least sixteen miles per hour and downing two bottles of sports drink, two bottles of water, and five or six gels, so that kept me busy trying not to drop my bottles or my gels. Then there was the pedaling, the passing, the being passed, the shifting of gears, and the avoiding of dead possums on the roadside. No time to be bored, and the scenery was magnificent. I was a little disappointed that at the turnaround at Pigeon Point, my average speed was only 15.9 miles per hour, but I hoped that the tail wind on the back half would help make up the time.

Oh boy, did it ever. I was flying. At the steep, straight downhill at Scott Creek, I crouched low over my handlebars and freewheeled down the grade, touching fifty miles per hour at one exhilarating point. I was having a ball, and my legs still felt pretty strong. I was trying to hold back a bit and conserve some leg power, since I was going to have to run thirteen miles afterwards. I didn't know my exact time for the bike leg as I hadn't taken careful note of my start time, but I knew I was going to be well ahead of schedule. Pretty soon we were back in town, bumping over the potholes and complaining about their effect on our butts.

A great thing about triathlons is having traffic blocked off for you. As I came screaming down the hill back onto Beach, I realized to my great delight that the intersection was all mine, thanks to the lovely police officers and their orange cones. I whizzed up to the dismount point with the volunteer hollering, *"Slow down!"* I *was* slowing down; it's just that I had been going quite quickly. I vaulted off the bike and jogged into transition, hollering to anyone in earshot, "Oh my god my butt hurts! oh my god my butt hurts!" Then I heard a familiar voice shriek, "Jayne!" Hey, it's Mom! Hi, Mom, my butt hurts. I was so stoked to see her there. Back to transition, get the socks on, ahhhh, and back out onto the road. There's Mom taking pictures, literally jumping up and down with excitement.

My legs didn't even feel that bad after the bike, considering. What I noticed very early on, though, is that someone had placed a balloon full of gas and rats inside my abdomen while I was focusing on the bike ride. With every step, my bloated belly made squirming motions and threatened to expand beyond its allotted boundaries. Also, I realized that I should have stopped to stretch my back and hamstrings for, say, an hour before heading out on the run. A few seconds here and there of putting my foot up on a handy bench and stretching out didn't really seem to do more than hold the stiffness at bay.

It wasn't bad enough to even consider quitting, though, so I just kept working on my rhythm and repeating, "I am relaxed and comfortable, I am relaxed and comfortable," even though it was a little bit of a lie. And I was having fun regardless. Michelle and Russ pulled up a few times in their car to wooo-hoooo at me and take unflattering pictures, there were SVTC members manning the aid station at the lighthouse, and it was a perfectly gorgeous day to run along the coast. We headed along the West Cliff path with the walkers, rollerbladers, surfers, dogs, and kids, until we turned up through a warehouse district and over the railroad tracks. This less-scenic bit led us to a lovely rolling bike path parallel to Highway One, where we toddled along for another couple of miles before Wilder Ranch Park. The five-mile marker came up and I realized that I had been feeling kind of OK for the last couple of miles.

Once into the park, I started to anticipate the much-vaunted Tiki Turnaround, the midpoint of the run. The race organizers had made a big deal of the Tiki Turnaround, so I was figuring there'd be hula dancers, music, drums, fresh pineapple, you know, a big party to boost our morale for the home stretch. My first disappointment was that the thing I thought was going to be the turnaround was actually just a regular aid station and it wasn't even at mile six—we had a mile-and-a-half loop to run before getting back to that aid station. Ergh. More steady trotting along. I was starting to walk the longer uphills as well as the aid stations but other than that, still feeling reasonably strong. The ol' stomach was still a little dodgy though—belching and passing gas were little moments of joy every time they happened.

At last I could see people turning around up ahead. The Tiki Turnaround was not a complete misnomer—it was in fact the turnaround, and there was a three-and-a-half foot tall Tiki god around which we had to run. One Tiki god and two dudes with plastic leis and sun hats, that's it. "*This* is the Tiki turnaround?!" I queried them. "I thought there'd be like music and hula dancers and that." "Would you like us to hula for you?" one of the dudes responded. "Yeah, that'd be good," I replied in all sincerity. So they got up out of their chairs and hula-ed for me for a little while as I jogged backwards along the path. It was good. I was energized.

But not for long. It was such a very long way back to the aid station, and then a long way again to the eight-mile mark. I became convinced that the eight-mile sign had been moved by malicious goblins, but it showed up eventually, and it was mostly downhill to the nine-mile, where Russ and Michelle were waiting for me with high-fives and more photo snapping. Only four miles to go! I was really starting to feel the exhaustion though. My stomach had more or less settled, but my body was just starting to ache all over, like a nasty case of the flu. On the downhills, even my fat hurt where it jiggled. My breathing muscles were aching, my back and shoulders and neck were aching, my legs were beyond aching. My walks through the aid stations started getting longer. When I stopped to walk and bend over and stretch, little whimpers escaped my lips. I did a bit of repeating, "I am comfortable and relaxed. I am at ease with this distance," and even though I knew full well I was lying like a rug, sometimes it helped.

Finally I got to the last aid station, where SVTC folks were still handing out water and cheering like crazy. I was so happy to see them I just wanted to cry. I turned the corner by the lighthouse and I could see the Boardwalk and the finish area, but I still had a mile to go. In other races this is where I pick up my pace for the finish and set my sights on catching or holding off some other competitor, but after almost six-and-a-half hours, there wasn't really anything left in the tank. Coming down the hill by the Dream Inn, I rolled off the path and onto the beach. It was like one of those nightmares where you're moving your arms and legs, trying as hard as you can to run, but you're just not going anywhere. The soft sand just sucked me in. I could barely stumble through it and onto the hard-packed sand by the water, but once I did, I actually did feel a little surge of energy.

Dodging toddlers and waves, I shouted out to folks on the beach, "Where the *hell* is the finish line?!" They pointed vaguely ahead at the wandering mob of people. Yes, but where's the line? The actual *line*? But before the line I saw my husband! Woo hooo! And Russ and Michelle—dang those guys get around—and my Mom! I turned off the hard pack onto the soft sand and saw a ledge in the sand looming in front of me. I had no idea how I was going to get up it. It must have been at least eight miles high. Or eight inches. Fortunately my Dad was there at the top of the ledge, and seeing him propelled me up and over the top. Only a few more feet, and I crossed the line. I cannot express how weary I felt, but when I hugged my Dad, I felt like leaning all my body weight on him was a really good idea. I would have fallen down on the sand, but I was pretty sure I wouldn't get back up any time soon.

I was showered with leis, hugs, pats on the back, bottles of water. I had completed my first half-Ironman. I was half an Ironwoman. The leis were scratchy so I took them off, went down to the water and walked in. The cold on my legs felt amazingly good. So I sat down. It was the best sixty-two-degree water I have ever felt. I floated, I moved my arms and legs around, I waved to my posse on the shore. I would have stayed there for a really long time but it was getting to be time for some real food. My stomach had pretty much returned to normal as soon as I stopped running, and it was letting me know that the oatmeal was a very long time ago.

So I am half iron. But which half? Maybe the upper half, 'cause the lower half sure didn't feel that great when the race was done. But my butt held up to the rigors of the bike ride pretty darn well, so maybe it's iron. And I didn't get even one blister on my feet, so they might be iron as well. They certainly were heavy enough to be iron. The bits of me that often chafe painfully? Chafe-free. Iron. My knees? Iron. My gut? Not iron. My quads? Not so iron. My lower back? Definitely clay, and crumbling clay at that. My skull must be iron, 'cause you gotta be pretty hardheaded to actually do this thing. So far my biggest endurance epics have been halfs. Half-marathon, half-Ironman. One of these days I have to do the other half of something. I'll wait for the swelling to go down on my right foot (maybe not iron after all?) and the memory of all the pain to recede before I think about that.

Oh, yeah—six hours, forty minutes, and twenty-three seconds. Right on the money for the goal I set myself back in February. Scary. And 3,749 calories burned up, according to my Polar A5 heart rate monitor. A good day's work.

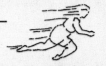

The Slow Fat Triathlete
Recommends

1. Don't be afraid to challenge yourself some more. You are mighty. You are a triathlete. You want to swim the English Channel? Go for it. Qualify for Kona? You da man. Do an Olympic distance tri? Yes! Figure out what you need to do to get to that place, and how long it will take to get there, and take your next step tomorrow. It could be that your next step is a day or two of recovery after finishing your first race. But that's an important step.

2. At the same time, don't feel pressured to do more or longer races right away. If all your training buddies are setting a goal of an Oly race in six weeks, and you just don't feel that you could do it without hurting yourself, then be smart. Back out and stay healthy. Maybe you'll be ready for the Olympic distance in three months, maybe next year. There's no rush.

3. Be curious. Find out what other kinds of events are out there. Find someone to train with you or to road-trip with you to a race out of state or out of the country. Enter some weird little open water swim race that you had never heard of before you entered the triathlon world. Dust off the mountain bike and do an off-road event somewhere.

4. Clubs can be fun—bike clubs, running clubs, swim clubs, open water swim clubs, trail runners, trail riders, other tri clubs. See what's going on with them. Maybe join your local chapter of the Hash House Harriers, "a drinking club with a running problem." You can learn new skills, get fresh perspectives, find new routes, meet new people.

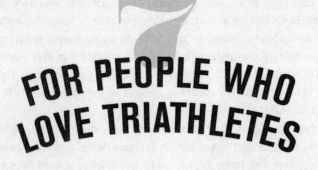

FOR PEOPLE WHO LOVE TRIATHLETES

HOW TO BE A TRI SUPPORTER

CHANGE OF PACE here, Mr. or Ms. Triathlete. For the last six chapters, it's been all about you. And me, of course, but there has been a lot about you. I've been blathering on about your physical training, your state of mind, your equipment, your schedule, your race day, and your plans for the future. Only rarely have I mentioned those loved ones who support you endlessly, from taking care of the kids to forgiving your exhausted crash into bed at 8 P.M. This chapter is for them. Hand the book over to your spouse or partner or significant other or mom and go find something to do with yourself for an hour. Stretching is always good.

Welcome, those who love triathletes. Your burden is heavy, but your rewards are great. You are blessed with a partner or family member who wants to challenge himself or herself, get more fit, have more fun, and blow a huge chunk of your family budget on equipment, race fees, club memberships, and probably therapeutic massage, too.

At the urging of my best friend Michelle, whose boyfriend Russ provided the catalyst for my plunge into the tri life, I'm including some tips on how to survive your loved one's new obsession.

PUTTING UP WITH THEIR TRAINING SCHEDULE

IT CAN BE extremely unnerving when your previously sluggish non-triathlete suddenly develops a training schedule and starts disappearing to the pool or the track or the road at all hours of the day and night. Household chores go undone, the lawn gets long and weedy, bills are left unpaid. It's not a pretty sight. In my case, however, the household chores, lawn, and bills were always extremely low priorities, and triathlon training just provides an excellent excuse to leave them way down on the list of things to do.

You may wish to point out to your budding triathlete that they should add to their training volume slowly and gradually. Going from zero hours a week to ten or fifteen can do more harm than good, especially for the previously inactive or currently tubby among us. Also point out the cross-training benefits of using pruning shears, raking leaves, or dusting bookshelves.

More importantly, you may start to feel like a triathlon widow or widower, and your kids may not recognize Daddy/Mommy when he or she finally rolls home. Your triathlete still loves you, rest assured. This is just something she has to do. It's a little bit of insanity that will lead to a greater sanity in the long run. In theory, as your triathlete gets fitter and gains confidence in her abilities, she will be a better person to be around, more complete, more energetic, more emotionally fulfilled, and a better partner and parent. And don't you want that for her? So you have to microwave a few dinners or trip over a pair of bike shoes. It's a small price to pay,

Another option is to join 'em if ya can't beat 'em. Bundle up the kids and go down to the track *en famille*. Your triathlete can run, you can walk, and the kids can play in the grass or the long jump sand pit. You could take up triathlon yourself, or at least part of it. Develop your long-stifled passion for cycling or running, or even swimming. We could all use a little more exercise, right?

And show your triathlete this paragraph: It's key to schedule date time or other non-triathlon fun time. Whether it's dinner and a movie or a weekend at the beach, the lake, or the mountains, your triathlete needs to recognize that you count, your relationship counts, and that part of your life together has to get on the calendar. For most of the triathletes I know, they've come to an understanding with their families about priorities, and workouts get scheduled in around family as a matter of course.

It's just that in the excitement of getting into a new sport or training for a big race, it's easy for the new triathlete to go overboard and schedule a lot of tri-stuff that doesn't include the important peeps in their life.

Fortunately, my husband is one of those guys who relishes time alone to play guitar and muse on the deep philosophical questions. Our psycho-kitty surrogate child is also fairly undemanding of my time. But I keep checking in with Tim on whether he's OK hanging out while I head out on a three-hour bike ride. Of course, he's usually fast asleep when I leave, so it's not like he notices.

PUTTING UP WITH THEIR NEW TOYS

IF YOU SNUCK a peek at Chapter Three while your triathlete was out training, you'd see that reading about triathlon equipment, talking about it, looking at it, shopping for it, buying it, cleaning it, and finding somewhere to put it are going to take over his life. Girls are just as bad in this regard. Hope you have a nice big garage.

I have three bikes at the moment, counting my trusty but space-consuming old recumbent, and Tim has one, which of course he never rides. We do not have a nice big garage, or a garage of any kind. A couple times a week I hear curses from the back patio as Tim trips over one of the bikes or my bike shoes or my pump or my stationary trainer, all of which are leaning against the back wall. Sometimes the wetsuit escapes the shelf above the washing machine in the utility room and lands on Tim's head as he pulls laundry out of the machine, or he can't get around the clothes rack where my workout clothes are drying on the patio. Then there's the bathroom where I store my sweaty garments until the next wash so they don't stink up the bedroom, the swimsuit drying in the shower, my running shoes all over the floor. Catalogs for bikes, bike parts, and workout wear, running shoes, triathlon-specific goodies, and swimsuits litter the coffee table and the floor. I know, it's a zoo, and he's a doll for only cursing a couple times a week.

And if you hadn't already noticed, this stuff costs money. Just think of all that cash as an investment in your beloved triathlete's long-term health. Of course, she's gonna be so healthy she'll outlive your retirement savings, already greatly depleted by outlays on tri gear. Hey, a custom-built carbon-frame feather-light max-aero tri bike is a pretty good inheritance to leave to your kids, right?

TALK TRI TO ME, BABY

SO YOU'VE ACQUIESCED to the inevitable—you're going to support your triathlete heart and soul. You're going to live with him waking you up as he leaves for pre-dawn workouts, leaving sweaty stuff everywhere, and spending all your money on things made of titanium. And you want to be able to talk to him, right? So here's a brief and extremely unreliable glossary of triathlon jargon that you can use so that you can conduct some kind of conversation about his obsession in the few minutes a week that you actually see each other. This can really enhance your relationship. I was so proud of my Mom—before my last race, she actually asked me, "What time do you think you'll be getting into T1?" It was a heartwarming moment.

AERO: short for aerodynamic. Most commonly applied to handlebars that allow a bike rider to get lower to the bike frame, decreasing wind resistance. You can also use this to describe any tapered-looking bike part, or to the position a rider is in, or to the bike itself, if it is sleek and shiny and looks extremely uncomfortable.

AEROBIC: the mode of exercise in which your muscles are getting enough oxygen to enable them to keep working for a long period of time.

AGE GROUP: In triathlons, you enter as a member of an age group, usually counted in five-year increments, e.g. twenty to twenty-four, twenty-five to twenty-nine, thirty to thirty-four, etc. The vast majority of people who participate in the sport are known as "age groupers," those who have no realistic shot at winning the race outright, but are in it for the fun, or maybe to come in the top ten of their age group. The age groups get a little smaller as you get older. If you're old enough, your age group shrinks to the point where you can win prizes just by doing the race. I'm not there yet, and I hope by the time I get there that the other old ladies will have had their fill of triathlon, leaving me with a hope for a podium finish. No, I'm kidding. My real dream is to see whole races full of fit, happy, seventy-year-old women out there doing triathlon with me.

AID STATION: the thing you long for during the run leg of a triathlon. Wonderful, kind-hearted volunteers hang out at tables with hundreds of cups of Gatorade and water and hand you fluids. Sometimes even energy gels and bananas. We love aid stations. They usually have them every mile or so.

ANAEROBIC: the mode of exercise where your muscles are not getting enough oxygen to fuel them. If you're sprinting, or riding your bike up a really steep hill, your heart rate goes up, you start to feel your legs burn, and guess what? You're in anaerobic mode. You can't keep this stuff up for very long. It hurts like hell.

ATHENA: race organizers' euphemism for female triathletes who weigh over 150 pounds. This cracks me up because I *dream* of weighing 150 pounds. At some races, you can enter as an Athena and then see how you do compared to other women who also happen not to be painfully thin.

BONK: what your triathlete's body does when it's out of gas. If she doesn't consume enough fuel when she exercises for a long time (more than sixty to ninety minutes), she'll run out of available sugar in her muscles and liver to keep herself going. Then she will feel yucky. Shaky, nauseated, weak, disoriented, all kinds of bad stuff. Make sure she takes sports drinks and energy gels out on long rides or runs.

BRICK: what you want to throw at your triathlete when he cleans his greasy bike on the living room carpet. No, not really. A brick is a training session that combines a swim and a bike, or a bike and a run. Bricks are often challenging, so offer props to your triathlete when he comes home from one.

CARBO-LOAD: the most fun part of pre-race preparations, involving eating massive amounts of pasta for three days before any event, no matter how short and insignificant. At least that's how I do it. I've even been known to carbo-load in support of my friends who are racing. If your triathlete's eating pasta, you eat pasta, too. (Actually, carbo-loading doesn't really help if the race is going to be over in ninety minutes or less, but it's so much fun and such a part of the tri tradition that I can't recommend against it.)

CLYDESDALE: another race organizer's euphemism, this one for guys weighing over 200 pounds. In my mind, a lot of Clydesdales are a lot more appealing to watch than these little 140-pound elf-boys who actually win the race. Some races have Lady Clydesdales. Oh yeah!

DRAFTING: the practice, usually illegal in age-group races, of getting your bike right behind the wheel of another bike in order to reduce wind resistance. If your triathlete says, "I got a two-minute penalty for drafting," console her. Here's the tricky bit, though—drafting is legal on the swim. You can tuck in behind someone's feet and save energy, if you know what you're doing, which I seem not to.

DUATHLON: a division of multisport where you run, bike, and run. Only two sports instead of three, hence "Du" instead of "Tri." I do not do the Du myself, 'cause I have more fun swimming than I do running, but you never know, one of these days.

ELITE: triathletes who have a chance of actually winning a race. These are often professionals as well as top-flight amateurs, and they have to take out special licenses and such. Also known as "the fast people."

EPIC: an adjective much overused to describe a training ride, run, swim or race that was some combination of long, hard, hot, hilly, windy, bumpy, or otherwise extremely challenging. Like I say, *Lawrence of Arabia* is epic. Your ride is only epic in your own mind. Use this word with caution, and if you hear it too much out of your triathlete, she may be in danger of taking herself too seriously, or she's been watching too much X-Games coverage on ESPN2.

FARTLEK: um, not what you think. This is a Swedish word meaning "speed play," and it's a kind of workout where you go faster for a while, and then go slower for a while. Like you might warm up, then run one minute faster, then two minutes slower, then two minutes a little faster, then a minute slower, and so on. The idea is to mix up your pace, give yourself a chance to experience a little faster speed, and then recover. From my perspective, "speed" is a misnomer anyway, but I do enjoy these kinds of workouts.

GI DISTRESS: gastro-intestinal distress. A useful catchall term for anything bad that happens to your gut region. Bloating, cramping, nausea, diarrhea, vomiting, all that good stuff all go into this category. Some people are really prone to this sort of thing, whether because of delicate stomachs, twitchy bowels, nervous dispositions, or a tendency to eat too much sugar on the bike and not drink enough water. The longer your race, the more of a danger this is. I was immune until I did a half-Ironman, and then that was just uncomfortable. Just one of the hazards.

HALF-IRONMAN: A race that starts getting into serious endurance, consisting of a 1.2-mile swim, a 56-mile bike ride, and a 13.1-mile run. There are people who tackle this distance for their first triathlon. I was not one of them, nor would I recommend it unless you already have serious experience with long-distance running or cycling or both. If your novice triathlete gets a wild hair and starts talking about starting off with a "half," discourage him gently.

HAMMER: to go hard for a sustained period of time, especially on the bike.

INTERVAL: another method of training/torture, involving working hard for a designated time or distance and then resting or recovering for another time or distance. So your triathlete might do eight hundred meters on the track at a moderate to hard pace (after warming up for ten to fifteen minutes, of course), followed by a minute rest, and repeat that four times. Interval training is one of the ways you can get a little faster and build your endurance in a pretty concentrated workout. Translation—intervals often hurt.

IRONMAN: the serious, serious distance. Swim for 2.4 miles, bike for 112 miles, and then run a full marathon of 26.2 miles. The first one was held in 1978 in Honolulu, and fifteen men participated. Now thousands of men and women compete in Ironman races from New Zealand to France to Wisconsin, but Ironman Hawaii, now held on the Kona coast of the Big Island, is the sport's holy grail.

NEGATIVE SPLIT: This is not when you take a look at a race course and go, "Oh, this totally sucks. I'm outta here." A negative split means doing the second half of your workout or race or race segment faster than the first half. This is usually a good thing 'cause it means you're pacing yourself well.

OLYMPIC DISTANCE: also known as international distance, a race with a fifteen-hundred-meter swim, a forty-kilometer bike, and a ten-kilometer run. (Just under a mile, just under twenty-five miles, and just over six miles is how we like to describe it in our metrically challenged country.) A nice distance for triathletes at all different levels. Sometimes shortened to Oly.

PRSS: Post-Race Stupidity Syndrome. It'll be obvious to you what this is after your triathlete's first race. Note that this is not a "real" piece of triathlon lingo because I made it up. I do believe, however, that PRSS is a widespread phenomenon and that this term will catch on pretty quick.

SPRINT: again, a serious misnomer as far as I'm concerned. Even the fast people don't finish these in too much under an hour. For me a "sprint" is something that lasts thirty seconds or less. Nonetheless, the sprint distance races, though they vary a lot, are usually around a four hundred-yard swim, a twelve-mile bike, and a three-mile run. I would highly recommend that your emerging triathlete do one of these for her first race.

SQUID LID: one of the greatest terms in all of sports, second only to "silly mid-off" which is something in cricket and therefore completely irrelevant here. A squid lid is a heavy-duty swim cap made of Neoprene and designed to keep your head warm in cold water.

STALL: a term for your little patch of ground in the transition area where you lay out all your stuff. I tend not to use this term as it has toilet connotations for me. And God forbid I should stoop to potty humor.

T1: the first transition of the race, from swim to bike. The part of the race offering the most opportunity for hilarity as dizzy, wet, cold, tired racers try and get out of their wetsuits and into their bike gear. Definitely take pictures here—your triathlete will so appreciate it.

T2: logically, the second transition, from bike to run. Not usually as entertaining as T1, although people do manage some funny maneuvers trying to get off their bikes at the dismount line.

TA: transition area-get your filthy mind out of the gutter! Besides, that's T *and* A. The transition area is where everyone sets up their bikes, gets prepared for the race, sets up all the gear they'll need for the bike and the run, and mills around chattering nervously.

THRESHOLD: where the pain starts. Also lactate threshold or anaerobic threshold. This is the point in training or racing where your triathlete is producing lactic acid in his muscles faster than his system can clear it out. This is because the body needs more oxygen to help make fuel for the muscles, and the level of effort is so high that he just can't metabolize any more oxygen. Training at levels of effort around your lactate threshold is very useful stuff.

WAVE: a moving bit of water. Also, confusingly, a group of triathletes about to jump in the water. Most races have "wave starts," where people go off at intervals to avoid congestion in the water. The first wave is usually the elites. Then the race organizers might send off all the men under thirty, then all the women under thirty, then men aged thirty to forty, and so on. The exact composition depends on the number of people in the race and the size of the start area. If your triathlete's wave goes off ten minutes after the first wave, the timing folks take that into account in the official results.

GOOD AND BAD THINGS TO SAY TO YOUR TRIATHLETE

NOW THAT YOU'VE got some of the vocabulary, we can work on using these words in sentences. We can also warn you about things not to say.

To make your triathlete feel fast, say, "You looked totally aero on your bike." Aero is good, but only on the bike. So don't say: "Dude, you looked so aero on the swim."

On hearing that the water temperature for an upcoming race is fifty-four degrees Fahrenheit: "Wow, are you going to need a squid lid for this race?" This demonstrates sympathy for the horrid conditions your triathlete will face in the frigid water. It also implies that you care about whether or not her brain freezes, and that brain freeze would be noticeable. So it's a good thing to say.

"What time does your wave start?" This demonstrates your understanding of the complex scheduling and logistical aspect of triathlon. It will also help remind your triathlete to check on what time his wave starts. It's soooo embarrassing to miss the start of your wave. You go tearing down the beach fumbling with your goggles yelling, "No, wait for me!!" Pathetic.

"You totally hammered up Nasty Grade!" Your triathlete will feel strong and fast, like a superhero, on hearing this description of her hill-climbing abilities.

Even if your triathlete manages to tie himself and his wetsuit together in an unsolvable knot during his swim-to-run transition, try and say something like, "Your T1 looked really fast." Don't say, "I didn't realize Neoprene bondage was one of the triathlon events."

If your triathlete asks, "Does this wetsuit make me look fat?" the correct answer is, "You look like a superhero!" Do not say, "Not compared to a bull sea lion."

And the number one thing *not* to say to your female triathlete, "Honey, how come all those gals in the Athena wave are skinnier than you?"

IT IS TOO A SPECTATOR SPORT

MY DEAR HUSBAND Tim very rarely comes to watch me race. His point, which is well taken, is that his experience of watching me race goes something like this: He has to get up early on a weekend, hang around before the start, watch the swim start as I disappear into a crowd of thrashing bodies, and then try and catch a glimpse of me as I emerge, dressed in the same black wetsuit and same color swim cap as everyone else in my wave. Then he races over to transition to watch me sail away on the bike. Then I'm gone for anywhere from one to three hours, depending on the race. Then he has to figure out timing and try to be alert to try and watch me coming in on the bike among hundreds of other whizzing forms. Then I slip on my running shoes, high-five him, and disappear again for an hour or two. If he misses me on the transitions, then many hours can pass between sightings. He finds it a little, well, boring, except for the few moments when I'm visible. And all the hanging around makes his back hurt. "It's not really the greatest spectator sport," he says.

Well, maybe not. But some people ignore Tim's clear-headed analysis and come out to watch anyhow. So if you do intend to venture out on race morning with your triathlete, here are a few observations and tips to up the fun factor for you.

RACE DAY FOR THE TRIATHLON SUPPORTER

WE HAVE TO make sure that you are prepared for all the likely eventualities with proper clothing, equipment, and nutrition. You will be armed with key information like when the race starts and when your triathlete's wave starts, and you will enhance your experience by cultivating certain key skills.

CLOTHING

Comfort above all else. Maybe you feel that your triathlete would get a real kick out of seeing you at the finish in your leather miniskirt and spike heels, especially if she hasn't seen you in that kind of attire before, but I'd recommend against it. You're going to be standing around, walking around, occasionally dashing from one spot to another, and probably sitting on the ground at some point. There aren't usually bleachers at triathlons.

Dress in such a way that you can be outside from before dawn through the full heat of the day and be comfortable. Where I live, it can be thirty degrees colder at 5 A.M. than it is at noon. And have some kind of hat to keep the sun off your head. An umbrella, perhaps, if you live in a place where it rains in the summer?

NUTRITION (YOURS)

Your triathlete has to be well fueled for optimum performance; likewise, you need to make sure your nutritional needs are taken care of for optimum fun as a spectator. I recommend one thermos full of coffee for the morning, and another thermos full of margaritas for when the sun warms things. Donuts for the morning, chips and salsa to go with the margaritas. Life is simple. Life is good.

The coffee actually is a good idea, if that's one of your drugs of choice. You may have to get to the race site absurdly early, and not all race sites sell coffee. The ones that do have an espresso stand do great business, but you may not know in advance whether you will be so lucky. Likewise with food. Quiz your triathlete about the race site and what sorts of amenities are nearby. You don't want to be stuck out on the course for several hours getting weak and faint from lack of food. When your triathlete finishes the race, the organizers will ply him with fruit, bagels, and sports drinks, but you, the dedicated support crew, will be out in the cold unless you can get him to sneak you a banana or two. Avoid being in this humiliating position. Carry your own snacks. And water. Hydration's important for you, too.

EQUIPMENT (YOURS)

You don't need the overwhelming pile of equipment that your triathlete does, but a few things may help your race day run smoother.

- **CELL PHONE** I don't encourage calling your triathlete while she's racing, but it's a good way to hook up after the race if you get separated in the crowd.
- **WATCH** For estimating your triathlete's arrival times on the different legs.
- **FOLDING CHAIR** You know those nylon/metal things that collapse into a tube and slip into a bag that you carry on your shoulder? Cheap and very handy, as triathlon courses tend to be pretty short on comfy chairs.
- **SUNSCREEN** That hole in the ozone layer ain't getting any smaller, last I heard.
- **CAMERA** For your role as race documentarian. We'll go into this in more depth later.
- **MAGAZINE** It might be a while between sightings of your triathlete. Reading material can be helpful, especially if you're a solo supporter. Crosswords are good.
- **BACKPACK** To carry the above, plus your food, water, coffee, and thermos full of margaritas.

BEING ABLE TO NAP IS GOOD

My friend Michelle often accompanies her long-time boyfriend Russ to races, especially if they're in pleasant locations like the Sonoma wine country or the beaches of Santa Cruz and involve an overnight at a charming country inn or even a Best Western motel. Sometimes her accompanying involves getting up at 5 A.M. so that Russ can get to the TA (remember TA?) in plenty of time to set up, get his number marked on his body, visit the Porta-John, get into his wetsuit, and get to the start. So she has cultivated her already prodigious talent for napping, catching a quick snooze in the car between the time they park the car and the time the race starts.

BEING CALM IS GOOD

Some triathletes get pretty amped up before the start of a race. Russ tends to appear calm, but he has his inner game face on, and his intense focus can affect his vocabulary and his judgment. The day before his first marathon, he held out a bunch of bananas and asked in all seriousness, "Would anyone like a balloon?" How we laughed! But Michelle loves to tell the story of how, on the way to his first half-Ironman, Russ realized that he had left his pump standing in the driveway. He erupted in a fit of swearing, cursing his stupidity and lack of attention to detail. "Where the f*** am I going to find a pump? Jesus Christ!" And here's where remaining calm is good: Michelle pointed out that they were heading to a triathlon, where every participant would have a bicycle, and many of them would even have bicycle pumps. It is a great credit to Russ's sense of humor that he is still able to laugh at this story.

The moral is that a supportive significant other ideally keeps a cool head when all about them are losing theirs. Tell them it will all be OK.

Even though he doesn't often come to races, Tim is very good at soothing my jangled nerves when I'm pacing the house the day before, wondering what I'm going to forget. He's also very good when I walk up to him with wild, staring eyes and go, "Aaaaaaaaah!" He knows just what I mean, and he stays very calm. "You'll do fine," he assures me, and I believe him. Or else he just opens his eyes real wide, too and goes "Aaaaaaaaah!" back at me, which cracks me up every time. So being calm is good the day before race day, even if you're not planning to go to the race.

BE A HOMEGROWN PHOTOJOURNALIST

One of your big roles as a tri supporter on race day involves documenting the entire day on film and/or video for the future glorification and/or embarrassment of your triathlete. This part of the deal involves long minutes or hours of inactivity as you wait for her to reappear, punctuated by a few seconds of frantic scurrying around to get a good shot in adverse circumstances.

Start capturing the day as early as possible. If you can get a good bleary-eyed 5 A.M. shot of your triathlete drinking coffee with one hand while trying to load the bike onto the car with the other, that sets the stage nicely. Take pictures of him getting body-marked, standing in line for the can, and other typical race-day adventures.

You'll want to try and get some kind of photograph of your triathlete at the start. This is a huge challenge. Unless you stick to her like glue, it'll be easy to lose her. She'll be wearing the same color swim cap as everyone else in her wave, she'll probably have one of the same four brands of wetsuit as everyone else, and she'll be wearing goggles. I swear to you I would not recognize myself in that get-up. In fact, I once got on the Internet and ordered a race photo of myself emerging from the water and peeling off my wetsuit, only to realize when the print arrived that it wasn't me at all. Getting shots of your triathlete emerging from the water poses the same challenge.

In Chapter Five I advised your triathlete to formulate a race plan. They should have some idea of how long it will take them to do each part of the race. If you coordinate those estimated times with your triathlete's wave start time, you may even be able to figure out when you need to be alert for him to show up. The biggest problem is he could be wrong.

Get a shot of the swim exit, then scurry quickly over to the transition area to get great wetsuit wrestling shots. Note that race organizers usually keep all non-racers out of the TA, so you'll have to hang over the fence as best you can to holler encouragement and wield the camera. Try and memorize what your triathlete's wearing, especially their top and helmet. This will help to identify them later. Once your triathlete takes off on the bike, scope out the transition area and the end of the bike course to see where you can get the best shots of your triathlete coming back in. Try to pick spots where your triathlete will look like he's moving fast. This will gratify his ego immensely. Downhills are good for looking fast, but unfortunately it also means you have to have quick reflexes to get a good photo as he goes zooming by.

Now you can relax for a while, hang out on your folding chair, read your magazine, drink some of your coffee. Check your watch and estimate when you need to be at your next photo spot. I can't overestimate the importance of checking with your triathlete on what times you think they'll be doing on the different legs. A fast cyclist might do a twelve-mile bike leg in around half an hour, while a velocity-challenged individual might take an hour or more. That's a lot of waiting around if you don't have an estimated arrival time.

A few minutes earlier than your earliest estimate, go to your photo spot. A lot of times people are too conservative in their estimates, not factoring in the adrenaline of race day. Cheer and wave and take photos as your triathlete passes, and scurry back to transition to stake a spot at the run exit. A hearty smooch might be just what the doctor ordered as your triathlete heads out onto the run course.

OK, you're both on the last leg of the race. Your triathlete's working a little harder than you are, but you may be getting tired, too. I think that watching a race is almost as tiring as doing one. Depending on the length of the race and the start time, you may find that now is the time to crack open that thermos of margaritas and start making some new friends out on the course. Or at least drink some water and eat a banana. You want to be feeling fresh and energized, or perhaps completely snockered, to get a hearty cheer going at the finish.

You will no doubt have studied the map of the run course, so you'll know whether or not it's an out-and-back, a big loop, or multiple loops. If there are multiple loops, you may get more than one glimpse of your triathlete. Otherwise, stake out a spot near the finish and get ready to make some noise.

Depending on your caffeine and/or alcohol intake and your natural level of enthusiasm, you may want to start cheering for all the finishers as they come in. They really appreciate it, believe me. There's nothing like a wave of noise to make a triathlete pick up his feet and try to look fast as he approaches the line, tongue hanging out from exhaustion. But of course, save your loudest holler for your own triathlete, of whom you are so very proud.

And don't worry too much if you didn't get good pictures. Most races have a photography service so you can buy a finish line photo and maybe even some other shots.

THE BIG FINISH

When your triathlete crosses the line, fight through the crowds who mill around the finish and give her an enormous hug, no matter how sweaty she is. It will wash out. Make sure she gets water right away, and keep her moving around so her legs don't stiffen up. If she looks like she might hurl, back off quickly. I have never actually hurled during or after a race, but some people do, and I always feel like I'm going to.

POST-RACE

Once the immediate exhaustion has subsided, it's good to get your triathlete over to the racers' refreshment table. It's not just my own native gluttony that makes me say this. The folks who study exercise and nutrition swear that eating within a few minutes of finishing a race is key to helping your muscles recover. Eat a banana after racing, feel less pain and stiffness tomorrow. It seems to work.

If there's a body of cold water near the finish—like the lake or ocean the swim was in—encourage your triathlete to go stand in the water for a few minutes. It can really help reduce inflammation in the legs. Feels good, too.

You'll notice that PRSS sets in pretty much immediately after the race. Your triathlete may feature a vacant stare, inability to concentrate, and extreme difficulty in making any decisions whatsoever. Food and fluids help somewhat, but time is the only real cure. Help your triathlete make his way back to transition and pack up his stuff. If the TA volunteers don't want to let you in, just explain that he's suffering from Post-Race Stupidity Syndrome and needs assistance in getting packed up. I myself have stood at my transition area for long minutes, just staring at the pile that needs somehow to get back into my race bag. PRSS leaves you without a clue as to how it all got in there in the first place.

Help your triathlete get some dry clothes on. I know, she knew how to dress herself this morning, but now she's very, very tired. And if you can help your triathlete by doing all the driving for the rest of the day, that would probably be very greatly appreciated.

The post-race meal is a highlight of race day for triathletes and support crew alike. We're not talking about the banana and half a bagel right after the race. We're going for an all-out, guilt-free chow down extravaganza. The sports nutritionists might not sanction this mighty bloat-fest, but it is really fun. By the time your triathlete has hydrated, snacked, soaked, packed up, changed, and gotten to the car, she will probably be just about ready to eat real food.

The truly sad thing is that doing triathlon is just not a license to eat whatever you want all the time, at least if you want food in the kinds of quantities and varieties that I want food. In one hearty meal, I can consume more than the calories I burn off by swimming a mile, biking twenty-five, and running six. But this topic is probably a whole other book, or at least another chapter. Go out, eat the post-race chow, and be happy with yourselves. You and your triathlete both done good.

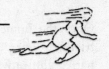

The Slow Fat Triathlete
Recommends

This sidebar comes in two parts, one for the triathlete, and one for the triathlete-lover.

FOR THE TRIATHLETE:

1. Remember to be extremely grateful to your spouse, family, friends, and co-workers who do whatever they do to support you. Even though triathlon looks like the ultimate individual sport, no one can really ever do it all by themselves.

2. If you use your training schedule as an excuse to slack on all your domestic responsibilities, this will rapidly become unpopular. Sometimes ya gotta suck it up and rake the leaves for an hour and ride your bike for an hour instead of hitting the autumnal roads for a nice long training ride.

3. Welcome your significant other's participation as a fellow athlete and/or spectator, but don't force it. If they don't want to ride bikes with you, just go out by yourself or find a training buddy.

4. Try and keep your sweaty workout clothes and gear in at least some kind of order. Pee-yew.

FOR THE TRIATHLETE-LOVER:

1. Figure out what's going to be acceptable and what's going to be a problem in the brave new world of having a triathlete in the house. Are sweaty socks really worth a battle? Maybe not. Disappearing for the

entire weekend, every weekend for training type activities? Yeah, I'd be ticked. Tell him or her what you need in order to make this thing work for both of you.

2. You may want to join in. What the heck, right? Get the whole family into it.

3. If you're a spectator, plan ahead for your own comfort and enjoyment. Drinks, food, folding chair, and the right clothes for possibly changing conditions.

4. You can take some really, really funny and embarrassing photos of your triathlete in action. Shots that will make your mutual acquaintances howl with laughter. Make sure you do this.

8

WHEN BAD THINGS HAPPEN TO SLOW FAT TRIATHLETES

INJURY, ILLNESS, OR
LOSS OF SENSE OF HUMOR

SO FAR THIS book has been all about the good stuff. Inspiration, motivation, accomplishment, animal joy in movement, the loyal support of your loved ones. The thrill of overcoming obstacles, stretching your limits, and chowing down guilt-free after a hard workout. (Again, DAIS, NAID—don't do this too often or the slow and fat will inevitably overshadow the triathlete. Sometimes a super burrito with the sour cream and guacamole is just what the doctor ordered, though.) But sometimes bad stuff happens to the best-intentioned triathletes. It's not all finisher's medals and sweaty hugs. You get hurt, you get sick, you get burned out, or, worst of all, you may lose your sense of fun.

That's the bad news. The good news is that with a very few exceptions, those things are temporary and you can keep on being a happy triathlete once time passes and you do the things you gotta do to get yourself better. The trick is that mental aspect of dealing with these setbacks can take as much grit and persistence as the mental side of training and racing, and it can be way harder to deal with than the physical pain. And sometimes, the smaller and sillier the injury seems, the harder it can be to stay patient and keep focused on your goals. I mean, if you break your leg, you know you have a serious thing going on and it behooves you to do exactly as your doc and physical therapist command to get it healed and rehabbed as soon as you can. But if you just have a pain in your hip that kind of comes and goes and you're not sure why, but some kinds of workouts make it worse, and the doctor can't really tell you what it is, and it goes on and on for weeks or months, that can be really hard to get through.

But you can get through it. You have to listen to what your body is telling you—and learn to interpret its vocabulary of tweaks, pulls, soreness, stiffness, strains, and sprains. And you have to keep your mind serene. A Tibetan Buddhist monk once instructed my friend Will that the secret of effective meditation was to "remain equanimous." Equanimousness, equanimity, thinking positive, whatever you want to call it, you'll need it. As I write these paragraphs, I'm feeling the aftereffects of a bike crash that's kept me on the couch all day and taken my Sunday long run right out of the equation. So I'm really speaking from the heart, yo. Ya feel me?

INJURIES

IN YOUR SPORTING life, you're going to see two kinds of injuries that affect people. You have your acute injuries, like an ankle sprain or a hamstring pull. Something happens to you, it hurts right away, you know you're hurt. The more insidious threats are usually the overuse injuries, where little traumas build up over time until you have a nagging pain in your knee or your heel or shoulder that sidelines you and derails your hard-won training discipline. Forewarned is forearmed, so maybe if I spend a few paragraphs on the most common hazards lurking below the happy surface of swimming, biking, and running, you'll exercise the eternal vigilance that is the price of injury-free triathletehood. And if you don't, I will come to your house personally and say, "What did I tell you?" as I pass you the Advil and ice pack.

ACUTE INJURIES

LIKE I SAID, these happen all at once. You're running along, you stumble over that raised patch of sidewalk, you turn your ankle. It hurts and then swells up like a balloon. You bang your knee on the edge of the pool and you get a horrific bruise, or if you're a little klutzy like me, you stub your toe on the leg of the coffee table and you walk funny for a couple of days. I'm not a doctor, or a physical therapist, or a personal trainer, or any of that. But there's some pretty commonly accepted wisdom on what to do for the bumps, bruises, and sprains.

RICE

IT'S ALL ABOUT the RICE. No, don't just cook up a big pot of rice and eat it with black beans. It stands for Rest, Ice, Compression, and Elevation. Stop using the injured part. Get an ice pack on it. You can get these nice gel packs that you can keep in the freezer for this sort of occasion, or you can use a bag of frozen peas. I would recommend using the same bag over and over, and not eating those peas. Write on them with a big black felt pen *"Therapeutic Peas—Do Not Consume"* and keep them in the freezer for emergencies. You can talk to twenty triathletes and get twenty opinions on your icing protocol, but I do twenty minutes or so, then wait an hour or two until the circulation's restored to the area, then ice it again. Do this until hypothermia sets in. Icing the injury is supposed to be best in the first twenty-four to forty-eight hours after you do it. It keeps the area from getting really inflamed and swollen. Elevation also helps with that nasty swelling thing.

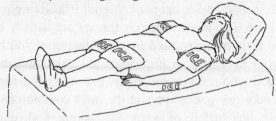

As for drugs, I say yes to them. Not anything illegal, of course (heaven forfend!), but your Advil, your Aleve, even your old-fashioned aspirin help with the pain, the swelling, and the inflammation. This is not the time to be stoic or Christian Scientific about taking a pill. The anti-inflammatories can really help you get back on your feet quicker.

If it's not significantly better in a few days, go to the doc. You might need some physical therapy and/or some better drugs. They might use ultrasound on the area, which provides deep heat to help promote circulation and get the swelling down, or electric stimulation, which tingles entertainingly and helps to control pain as well as getting the circulation going.

Another category of acute injuries is the bike crash. If you're careful and keep your equipment in good order and have a little luck, it could be years and years before you crash your bike. Until last Saturday, I hadn't taken a tumble in about eleven years. But if it does happen and you get a little banged up, a lot of the same tips apply. Ice the things that are bruised and take your Advil. You'll also have to clean up any road rash you may have acquired. It's good to do this as soon as possible after you fall, before it really starts to sting. Make sure you (or a helpful partner) can get all the dirt and gravel out. Now, again, there's a lot of controversy about what to do once you have it cleaned. A friend of mine, a former bike racer, swears that you need to keep the wound covered and plastered with Neosporin. Some people say you have to leave it exposed to the air, others say you should cover it with a flexible wound cover like Second Skin and *not* use an antibiotic ointment. I cover what I can and leave the rest.

OVERUSE INJURIES

THESE ARE THE ones that really get me. Odd pains in your feet or your knees, your hips, your lower back, your shoulder, whatever. There are so many ways that things can get sore, and I don't have any qualifications to tell you about them in any detail. However, I don't have any qualifications to write this book either, other than being a slow fat triathlete myself. So I'll tell you about a few of the common ones.

The key to avoiding overuse injuries is to avoid overusing whatever it is. Sounds easy, but if it really was, wouldn't we all be doing it? When you get started exercising, you're really vulnerable to overuse because you're going from basically no use to a bunch of use. It's like you have a car that's been sitting on the street for five years, hasn't had the oil changed or checked, the belts are all dried and shrunken, all the fluids are congealed, the moving parts are rusted into place—get my picture here? And then you take that car and you start it up and you tear off down your street at eighty miles an hour, belching blue smoke and back-firing like crazy. Would you even consider doing that to your car? Not if you wanted to drive it across country later in the summer.

No, if you were a responsible car caretaker, you would check out the car first, change out all the fluids, the spark plugs, the belts and all. You'd flush the radiator and then you'd take the thing out for an easy spin around the block, listening with all your attention for any odd sounds, sniffing the air for suspicious smells, using your body to feel any undue vibrations, watching for smoke or steam.

And, now that I've carried this heavy simile about as far as I can, I will point out that you should exercise at least that much care with your body when you start training for a triathlon or planning to do a 5K walk. You should always spend the first ten or fifteen minutes of any exercise session warming up real easy. Think of this as getting the oil distributed around your engine. As your muscles gradually get warmer, they relax and become more resilient, more resistant to injury. When they're cold and stiff, it's a lot easier to put small or large tears in the tissue. Over time those tears add up and you can end up with an overuse injury.

You also need to add to your exercise program in very small increments. Embarrassingly small. Pushing too hard too fast is a prime way to get hurt. Your joints and ligaments need time and a gradually increasing workload to get them toughened up. Your body can learn and adapt to changes in your habits, but it can't do it in a week.

I've said this before, too, but you can stand to hear this again: Stretch. Stretch when your muscles are warm—after you're done exercising and cooling down a little. If you try stretching when you're cold, the muscles are stiff, they're not stretchy, and they're vulnerable to getting hurt.

The bigger you are, the older you are, and the less athletic background you have, the more it will behoove you to be super careful about avoiding injury. Every little pound of extra avoirdupois you carry translates into extra stress on the joints, the muscles, the connective tissue. But if you insist on charging ahead full steam, taking on a hard workload right away, and not stretching, here's what you might have to look forward to, starting from the ground and working up:

▶ *Plantar Fascitis* A technical-sounding name for pain in the foot. "Fascitis" is inflammation of the fascia, a web of tough, thin tissue that holds your muscles and ligaments in place around your skeleton. Think of it as shrinkwrap around your meat. Down in your foot the fascia can get really tight, especially around the heel, that being a sort of fulcrum for the forces in your lower leg when you run. So you feel pain right at the bottom of your heel. Like a lot of overuse injuries, the place you feel the pain is not necessarily where the root of the problem is. If your calf muscles are tight, that can pull on the fascia in the foot and that's where you feel the pain. So a good way to prevent this injury is to keep stretching your calves.

▶ *Achilles Tendonitis* This is another injury that may well happen to you if you don't stretch the calves. The calf muscles end in this thick, gnarly tendon that's the biggest tendon in your whole body. It's big and thick because it has to spring your entire body weight off the ground when you walk or run. And the tendon—like tendons in general—can't have much stretch in it, or it won't do its job of providing leverage. So the muscles that the tendons are attached to have to have the stretch instead.

▶ *Patellar Tendonitis* Same deal, except it's the front of your knee that hurts, and it comes from your hamstrings being too tight, as well as your calves. Your patella is your kneecap, the rather loosely attached hockey-puck-like bit of bone that I always fear is somehow going to go astray under my skin and end up down my shin somewhere. The patellar tendon is the main thing that connects it to your shin bone. Am I getting this right? Must go check anatomy book. Hold on. Yup, that's right. A big old thick tendon that attaches to the top of your tibia, or shin bone. It's hard to explain why the lack of flexibility in the back of your thighs leads to pain in the front of your knee, but that's the complexity of the human body for you. Everything is interconnected. When your hamstrings are tight, it puts extra strain on your quadriceps in the front of your thigh. Then that pulls up on the patella, straining the tendon at the bottom of the kneecap and giving it these nasty little tears that lead to pain. You have to rest this until the pain goes away when you run or bike.

▶ *Iliotibial Band Syndrome* Big owie. The iliotibial band is this long, flat muscle that goes from your hip bone down the outside of your thigh and attaches to the top of your tibia, or shin bone. It does a lot of work stabilizing your hips and knees, and it gets really tight in most runners and cyclists. When it gets too tight, you can get pain in the outside of your knee and you won't know why. It can be really hard to stretch the ITB, too. It's tough to get the right angle. One of the best ways to do it is to roll the outside of your leg along a foam roller. These foam thingies are getting really popular in Pilates classes and physical therapy. They're usually about three feet long and about six inches in diameter, made out of a very firm foam. (Firm foam. Firm foam. Firm foam. I like saying that.) You can use them to roll out sore spots in your back, your hips, your butt, and your legs. They're awesome. You can get them from your local yoga or Pilates studio or online.

▶ *Piriformis Syndrome* A pain in the butt. The piriformis is a small muscle that runs horizontally along the back of your hip bone, underneath your big ol' buttock muscles, the gluteus maximus, medius, and minimus. It's another stabilizer and it also works to rotate your hips outward, like if you were going to point your toes out to the side. If your glutes aren't strong enough and you don't stretch regularly, your piriformis has to work too hard, and guess what? It tightens up. You may feel it as a pain in the ass, or your lower back may go out from the excess tension on one side of your hips. Another great use for your foam roller.

▶ *Rotator Cuff Issues* Pain around the shoulder joint, probably brought on by too much swimming with too little preparation, swimming with a flawed technique, or sometimes just by bad luck with your anatomy. Your shoulder has the widest range of motion of any joint in your body, thanks to an array of muscles that wrap around the bones, allowing your arm to move forwards, back, up over your head, out to the side, and all those other good directions. Swimming freestyle gives your shoulders the chance to get out and experience pretty much that whole range of motion, including some of the motions that can be a little bit of a strain, like reaching straight over your head as far as you can. When you do that, you risk getting some of those muscles, especially the supraspinatus on the back of the shoulder, pinched in the movement of the joint. Or you can just wear on one of the muscles with the unaccustomed repetitive motion of swimming. So work up really slowly with your yardage. Always swim easy for ten minutes or so before really trying to churn up that water.

▶ *Sore Neck* If you're not used to bicycling, and/or your bike's not adjusted properly, you might develop stiffness or pain in the neck. Actually, you want to know the real story behind how I write this stuff? I just wait for my next training injury to crop up and then I write about it. I had just gotten over my little bike wreck when my neck seized up two mornings ago as I stepped out of the shower. Now I don't know if that was to do with the falling off the bike, or with the crappy mattress Tim and I have been sleeping on for the last seven years, or something I did wrong at the gym. But I can tell you with white-knuckled sincerity that it hurts. My ace chiropractor/physical therapist tells me that one reason that this happens is that the front side of me is hunched over from too much sitting at the computer and riding my bike and not enough time stretching out my shoulders and pectoral muscles. Also, the scalenes, at the front and sides of your neck, get really tight from the kind of sitting-down, bent-over lifestyle that most of us enjoy. So get your pecs stretched out and your scalenes loose and don't stick your head forward when you sit at your computer.

LOSS OF SENSE OF HUMOR

WHAT MORE TO say? This is the worst disaster that can befall you. If your sense of humor wears out, the whole world of triathlon loses its silly glow. Trotting around the track while the greyhounds pass you changes from an amusing exercise in humility and self-discipline to a humiliating torment. The gigglesome feeling of your fat jiggling around your hips as you run turns into another humiliating torment. The self-indulgent warmth of nursing a minor injury over the weekend turns into a (humiliating) torment of self-flagellation: "Why didn't I take better care of my knee/ankle/foot/shoulder/back? I must be hurt because I'm so old/fat/out of shape/inflexible/female/male/impatient/lazy."

I think the root cause of this malady is the invidious practice of comparing yourself to other people. That person is faster than you. That other person or whole crowd of people is thinner than you. Other people are out there swimming, biking, running, or racing while you're at home nursing your sore toe. You are what you are right now. When the rosebud is still forming a little green ball, do you berate it for not being in full bloom? Hell no!

Stress and fatigue can also contribute to losing your sense of humor, or misplacing it temporarily. Your boss is emulating Saddam Hussein, one of the kids has the flu, and you're either feeling guilty about skipping your workouts or squeezing them in with grim determination. It ain't no thang if you need to blow off a training session or two. Presumably your family is more important than triathlon, as is your job—well, you sort of have to keep it to pay the bills. Now, I do find that a nice vigorous workout does wonders to help keep the stress in check. On the other hand, sometimes a nice hot bath at night and an extra hour in the sack rather than a trip to the spinning class is really what you need, physically, mentally, spiritually, and every other way.

WAYS TO KEEP YOUR SENSE OF HUMOR

SCHEDULE "NON-SERIOUS training sessions" with friends. Ride your bike to a donut shop and back. My tri club schedules a ride every fall that revolves around a massive brunch at Zelda's on the pier in Capitola. It's really hard to ride home 'cause it's all uphill and your gut is chock full of eggs Benedict, but it's worth it for the bonding experience.

Get someone to take a series of pictures of you putting your wetsuit on. When you feel gloomy, go back and look at them. Guaranteed chuckles.

Make a list of the top ten funny things about your working to become a triathlete. Might look something like this:

10. My training diet includes CinnaBons.
9. I would rather tattoo my own behind with a toothpick than go for an early-morning run.
8. There's no perceptible difference between my warm-up jog and my finishing sprint.
7. My swim stroke reminds onlookers of the *Titanic*.
6. I'm a forty-year-old cubicle slave with a secret triathlete alter ego.
5. For the amount of money I've spent on this suffering, I could have sprung for a week at the Kona Village resort.
4. My husband worries about me injuring myself putting on my wetsuit.
3. The only way I could ever qualify for the Ironman World Championships is by living to the age of ninety-five and winning my age group.
2. I can train twelve hours a week and still gain weight.

And, the number one funny thing about me becoming a triathlete:

1. *I'm a triathlete anyway!*

So there. Your setbacks are temporary. Your obstacles are just there to make it all a better story. Your physical and mental limitations are just part of the package. Go out and sweat, but don't sweat it.

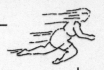

The Slow Fat Triathlete
Recommends

A few hints to keep your corporeal self and your spirit healthy and happy.

1. Warm up slowly. No matter what the workout, no matter how little time you have to get it done, warm up for ten minutes at an embarrassingly slow pace. Don't worry what anybody thinks of you, ever, and especially when you're warming up.
2. Stretch, stretch, stretch. Stretch like a rubber band. Stretch like Gumby. Take fifteen minutes every day when you would otherwise just be plopped in front of the tube and stretch. I like to plop on the floor in front of the tube and stretch then. Get up from your desk at work and stretch your back and your hamstrings for a minute or two.
3. Learn where your weak points are. A few weeks of training will probably make them pretty obvious. Maybe your neck gets sore on the bike, or your calves get tight, or your shoulder hurts from swimming. Then research how to fix that problem and work on it. Go easy on the weak bits—rest them when they hurt, stretch them gently or ice them or both—just not at the same time.
4. Epsom salts rule! When you have muscle soreness and aches and pains, pour a couple of cups of Epsom salts into a hot bath and soak until you're a limp noodle. These things really, truly work for reducing the soreness. The best explanation I've been able to figure out on the Internet is that the magnesium in the salts is absorbed through your pores and helps your muscles relax, which helps your body flush out the toxins that make you sore, while the sulfates in the salt are good at attaching to those toxins and making them easier to get rid of. Whatever the reason, it works and it has the added appeal of being extremely relaxing.
5. Forgive yourself and your body. It's never worth beating yourself up for getting injured or for skipping a workout. Regrets suck. Almost literally. They suck the life and the joy and the hope for the future right out of you and replace those things with a big pool of yuck.

9

ACTUALLY, YOU CAN'T EAT WHATEVER YOU WANT

THE SAD TRUTH ABOUT
TRIATHLON TRAINING

PEOPLE—ACTUALLY, WOMEN-type people—say to me all the time, "Whoa! You do triathlons?? You must be able to eat whatever you want!" To which I reply: "You have no idea how much I want." This is perhaps the saddest truth about triathlon for me. My body is not yet capable of training enough to burn off all the calories I would eat, given free rein. Even when I was training for a half-Ironman, I didn't lose weight. I got leaner, as I gained some muscle and lost some fat, but my net weight didn't really change.

There are lots of books out there about nutrition for endurance athletes, and about eating to lose weight, and of course the whole diet book mega-industry. The real key, though, to getting thinner and staying thinner, is that on average, you have to consume fewer calories than you expend. And that's incredibly hard for people like me who love French-fried anything, anything with extra cheese, and chocolate everything.

Take a typical workout for me. I might go out on my bike and ride for ninety minutes About twenty minutes of that is an easy warm-up, and the last fifteen minutes or so I cool down. In the middle I work pretty hard, hills or sprints or whatever. I work up a good sweat, and my average heart rate might be around 130. My heart rate monitor tells me I burned 478 calories. Cool! That should earn me the right to stop by the mall and buy one of those warm, gooey, yeasty, delicious CinnaBons, right? Nah. Those things are 730 calories apiece, and if you get the pecan ones, you're up to 1,100. And here's the thing—I can easily eat two of those things in a day. Just a little snack. Super size fries at McDonald's? 610 calories. And that's just the fries. Add in your Big 'n' Tasty with cheese, another 590 calories. Even assuming that you, like me, then order the Diet Coke, you're still in a deep caloric hole with that one meal, even though you worked out for an hour and a half.

Are you with me? Does this suck, or what? I want to eat more than I can burn off. I haven't figured out how to say *no* on a regular enough basis to lose the thirty or so pounds of fat that still cling to my frame in spite of four years of hard work, training, and watching my food intake most of the time. I don't really have the answer to this yet. If I did, I'd be writing *Moderately Fast Skinny Triathlete* instead. And would you buy that? Probably not.

If you're looking at this book as a path to weight loss, I have to tell you there ain't no easy road. You can get a lot fitter without losing a lot of weight, and that's a fine thing, too, if that's what you want. Me, I'm tired of jiggling when I run and I'm working on getting my weight down further. But I still want to enjoy food, enjoy dinners out, and have a good time. How to do that?

JUST EAT LESS

I LOST A bunch of weight on my own, pretty much by eating a lot less for breakfast and lunch, eating a moderate dinner, and cutting way back on dessert. I basically ate an energy bar, like a Balance Bar or Clif Bar for breakfast, and another one for lunch, with a few veggies thrown in. I was also exercising about an hour a day, aerobics, weights, cardio machines, kickboxing, lots of good stuff. I ate more vegetables and fewer potatoes, kept cheese and fried crap to a minimum most of the time, and drank very little alcohol. That helped me to take off about seventy-two pounds in under two years.

I won't say that it was easy, but it was my primary focus. Almost every single day was about losing weight. If I was really hungry going to the step class at the Y, so much the better, as long as I didn't pass out. I was exercising for weight loss, not for performance, so I wasn't worrying about fueling my workout.

This regimen took a lot of mental energy, and, frankly, I was hungry a lot of the time. After my wedding, though, I relaxed into that married bliss and started to lose my edge. I was also working in a company full of young guys who loved to eat cheeseburgers, pizza, donuts, and giant burritos, and I got caught up in their dietary habits. I had thought that in two years of work I had taught myself how to manage my food intake and my exercise, that I had changed my eating habits permanently. Wrong! Neither my ability nor my desire to inhale a bacon-smoky-cheddar burger and a huge basket of fries had diminished one whit. What had diminished was my ability to make up for a meal like that with a few days of light eating and plenty of veggies. Boom! I packed on twenty-four pounds in one short year.

WEIGHT WATCHERS

SO MY DOC suggested Weight Watchers. I was all, "Oh, doood. Weight Watchers is for like, my mom and her friends. Weight Watchers is so not cool." So I didn't go right away. But I kept getting fatter, and I finally decided that being fat wasn't necessarily real cool either. Much to my delight, it turned out that the Friday morning Weight Watchers meeting I picked at random was packed to the gills with smart, generous, insightful, funny women (and the occasional funny guy). Some had already lost their weight and were working on maintaining it, others were just starting or in the middle of a long haul. That Friday morning meeting is still a highlight of my week. The socializing rocks, and every week someone says something that stays with me and helps keep me at least somewhat motivated to get control of my eating habits.

The idea behind the current incarnation of Weight Watchers is that no food is forbidden, as long as you stay within your allotment of points for the week. You're also supposed to eat your five fruits and veggies every day, get calcium and protein in, and favor whole grains over white flour. Oh, and limit dietary fat. How could I forget? So it's basically eating a balanced lower-fat diet and keeping control of your portions. Having said that, if you want to eat a Krispy Kreme (six points for original glazed) instead of your oatmeal (one cup equals two points) every now and then, or even every day, you can do that, as long as you balance it out and stay within your points. Exercise is optional, but recommended, and the Weight Watcher is also urged to drink lots of water. It's just so darn sensible.

Weight Watchers also gives you some techniques for dealing with life in your food-centric world: office potlucks, holidays, vacations, pushy relatives, and so on. You get to practice techniques for getting to your goal, too—determining what you want in your weight loss efforts, why you want it, and how you're going to get there. Or mentally practicing saying, "No, thanks, I'll pass on the pecan pie." I've traditionally been skeptical of mental exercises like this, but I think they're actually pretty helpful. The same techniques work pretty well for me with regard to training and racing, so why shouldn't they work in my struggle with my food demons?

I'm still struggling, but I've lost thirty-five pounds with Weight Watchers and I'm at least addressing some of the ways in which my urges to eat are antithetical to my urges to be leaner and more fit. I'd recommend it to anyone with weight to lose, which is, again, pretty much everyone. And no, they're not paying me to say that. But if they wanted to, we could certainly talk about it . . .

Anyone who remembers the old Weight Watchers should be aware that it really has changed for the better. There is a great collection of Weight Watchers recipe cards from 1974, posted on the Web by a funny and subversive writer named Wendy McClure. Recipes include "Fluffy Mackerel Pudding" and "Jellied Tomato Refresher." Check them out at http://www.candyboots.com/wwcards.html, then go to Weight Watchers and be thankful it's not like that anymore.

BACON, BREAKFAST OF CHAMPIONS?

I KNOW A lot of people out there are doing the Atkins thing. Fat good, protein good, carbs bad. I also know it works for a lot of people. Some researchers at Stanford and Yale have decided that low-carb diets probably work because you end up eating fewer calories than you did before and you stick with it longer because you get to eat more fat, and possibly because your appetite gets suppressed when you eat this way. Other researchers say no, these very-low-carb diets don't work long-term.

I don't know how well it works when you're working out. Your liver transforms the carbohydrates that you eat into a sugar called glycogen, which is then stored in your muscles, packaged in water. When you exercise, your body taps into that glycogen for fuel. Conventional sports nutrition wisdom indicates that you then need to eat more carbohydrates in order to replace that glycogen. However, a couple of researchers have analyzed a lot of studies on Atkins-type diets and here's what they say about it:

> Several studies have shown that chronic consumption of very-low-carbohydrate diets leads to several metabolic and hormonal adaptations that facilitate increased fat oxidation and promote a glycogen-sparing effect within muscles.
>
> The effects of a very-low-carbohydrate diet on prolonged exercise performance are unclear; studies have produced inconclusive results. Although high-carbohydrate diets have historically been considered superior to high-fat diets for this type of exercise, studies have shown that very-low-carbohydrate diets may result in improved or maintained endurance exercise performance."
>
> (Volek, J. S., Westman, E. C., "Very-Low-Carbohydrate Weight-Loss Diets Revisited," *Cleveland Clinic Journal of Medicine*, 69(11), 2002, pages 849–862.)

What I think they're saying is that eating lots of fat and some protein and almost no carbs may somehow train your body to use fat for fuel rather than depleting the glycogen stored in your muscles, and that you may be able to be an endurance athlete and do Atkins.

Everyone's metabolism is different, too. I know people who seem to thrive with fewer carbs, and others who get so irritable that you want to run for cover. None of the sports nutrition experts whose words of wisdom I read in books, magazines, or online recommend Atkins, but if it works for someone, I'm not going to be the one to tell them that they're wrong. Let me know if it works for you. I'm curious. Dubious, but curious.

JUST EXERCISE MORE

YOU MAY BE at that delicate balance point with your metabolism and your weight where just adding exercise to your life could start you dropping pounds. If you aren't actively putting on weight at a rapid rate, and you don't currently exercise, this could work for you. Exercise gets your metabolism revved up so you burn more calories even when you're not exercising, which is cool.

EATING AND TRAINING

I'VE GOT TWO really big challenges going on with food and training. One is that I just love rich, high-calorie food. If I lived the arduous life of a hunter-gatherer in a difficult climate, my drive to find and consume fattening food would help me survive famine. However, I live in suburban California, where fattening, tasty food is everywhere and famine is not so much of an imminent danger. So being a fat-lover's not such an evolutionary advantage at this stage in America's development.

The other issue is that I find it hard to time and judge my eating so that I have enough energy in my bod to get through my workouts, without eating so much that I gain weight. For example, as I write this it's about 5:15 P.M., and I have to go to a pretty strenuous track workout at 6:15 and work out for about an hour. I ate lunch at about one, so now I'm pretty darn hungry. If I eat a handful of baby carrots and a few cucumber slices, I'm going to be so dizzy and weak at 7:00 that I won't be able to get the maximum benefit out of my training session. I can only imagine how athletes with diabetes figure out their eating and blood sugar and all that on a daily basis—it's complicated stuff for me just to figure out when I should snack so I won't get kind of irritable and feeble. So anyway, I'm chewing on a Clif Bar, which has lots of carbs and protein and vitamins and will sit OK on my stomach. But that's 250 calories, and a good chunk of my daily Weight Watchers' points allowance. It gives me pretty much no leeway for after-dinner snackage or other indulgence.

If you read other triathlon books, and I hope you will, they'll devote a lot of pages to the optimum balance of carbohydrates, protein, fat, and all that stuff for people who are training and racing. Some people will inveigh against refined sugars or potatoes or white rice. Others will urge you to eat as many whole grains and high-fiber meals as possible, except while actually exercising, when you should take in carbohydrates in the form of sports drinks or gels.

If you haven't been active and then start an exercise program, you may well start changing the way you eat. You may find that your traditional afternoon Cheetos and a Coke leave you feeling weird before your after-work training session. Or you may find that you need to start eating breakfast because you can't swim well without a little something in your stomach.

Experiment with what works for you and use common sense. Don't go into a workout feeling desperately hungry. On the other hand if you have to start your workout in twenty minutes, that is not the optimum time to inhale two slices of pepperoni pizza. Try something like a banana, or a NutriGrain bar, or a piece of toast. When you do eat a big meal, eat it at least an hour and a half before a training session or a race. It seems to be pretty widely accepted that a meal with protein and high fiber from veggies and/or whole grain products is going to give you more sustained energy than a mound of potatoes. Just make sure you give it that time to digest.

Surely I don't have to point out that from an overall nutritional standpoint, lean proteins, fresh vegetables and fruits, and whole grains are probably going to make you feel and perform better than chips, cheeseburgers, and donuts. That is, however, entirely up to you and what your goals are. If you can be a burger-hound triathlete, more power to ya. I wish I could be one, too. And most importantly, don't obsess about everything you eat, even if you are trying to lose weight and improve your fitness, unless that kind of obsession is rewarding for you. Life's too short and complex. What one nutritionist or coach recommends on her Web site might not work for you anyway. Everyone's metabolism is different.

A WORD ABOUT TRANS-FATTY ACIDS

THESE THINGS ARE the new bane of our existence. Refined sugar and even cholesterol are receding into the mists of former media frenzies now that partially hydrogenated fats, which contain the dreaded trans-fatties, have all the attention. Certainly they do seem scary. They raise your levels of bad cholesterol, lower your levels of good cholesterol, and, nastiest of all, they pretty much seem to attach to the walls of your arteries and stick there like Velcro. One nutritionist who consults for our tri club says unequivocally: "Trans fats are the only substance I recommend that nobody ever eat." He has strong opinions. The American Heart Association says to limit your saturated fat and trans fats to 10 percent of your total calorie intake.

The devil of it is that the partially hydrogenated fats are in pretty much every commercially available baked or fried goody. Triscuits? Loaded with 'em. Potato chips? Fuhgeddaboudit. Store-bought cookies, pies, frozen pound cakes, they are all just packed with those babies. They help stabilize the fat for longer shelf life. The folks who make these foods just don't understand that at my house none of that food needs to have a long shelf life. I don't really know what to do about it. The more I avoid those snacks, the better my weight loss efforts go, but sometimes I just give in and eat them anyway. Of course, you can make those yummy things at home, putting nice fresh butter and oil in them instead of these weird trans fats, and then they're even more tempting. But better for you. Unless you eat the whole batch at once, which I tend to. And who knows—maybe in ten years or so we'll learn from the science folks that it wasn't the trans fatties that were causing the problems after all, it was some other damn thing.

SPORTS DRINKS, GELS, ENERGY BARS

I TOUCHED ON this a little bit in Chapter Three, but it bears repeating: There's a whole boatload of different nutritional products out there that purport to help you exercise better. From Gatorade to Hammer Gels to G-Push with galactose, probably none of this will do any damage. And when you're working out for more than an hour, it will almost certainly help to consume some kind of sports drink or gel or something, either right before you start or after a half hour or so, or both. Otherwise you may run out of stored fuel in your muscles and you may feel kind of bad.

Believe it or not, there are actually techniques for drinking and eating these things. If you're doing a sports drink, start drinking as soon as you start exercising, in small quantities. When you eat a gel, wash it down with four to eight ounces of water. The gels are highly concentrated food, and you need the water so that your digestive system can actually process them.

NO CURE?

IS THERE A cure for being a chronic overeater? I'm still working on that one. Some weeks I'm on top of my game with the food thing, other weeks it's just a cavalcade of cookies. But I think for me the main thing is to be vigilant. I can't go on eating whatever I want to eat and pretending to myself or anyone else that I can just work out a little more to burn it all off. Not unless I change what I want. And I'm working on that, too. What does the future hold? Next year will I be writing *Moderately Fast Skinny Triathlete*? Or will it be *Still Kinda Slow, Still Kinda Fat*? I don't have a prescription for you to follow to manage your weight or change your eating habits. It's just like doing a triathlon, though. If you want to do something about where you're at, the key is to take a stab at it, start slow, go easy on yourself, and keep plodding along.

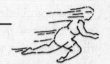

The Slow Fat Triathlete
Recommends

1. Decide What You Want. Are you interested in changing your diet along with your exercise habits, or are you pretty happy where you're at?

2. Start Small. If you do want to go from junk food processing machine to paragon of nutritional perfection, don't try and do it all at once. Start out by substituting a banana for your afternoon Twix, or eating whole grain cereal instead of the breakfast burrito. Do that for a couple of weeks and then find another thing you can change.

3. Read the Labels. Oh my God. It's amazing how many calories and fat are in the most innocuous-seeming things. If you're going to eat the thing, eat it, but face up to what you're eating.

4. Go Easy on Yourself. Just like your training, if you blow it one day, don't give up and don't give yourself a lot of grief over it. One snack or even one meal won't mean the end of all your hard work—unless you let it slide into another meal, or a whole weekend, or a week, or a month . . .

5. When in Doubt, Eat Vegetables. As long as they're not deep fried in batter or covered in cream sauce.

10

IN WHICH I TELL YOU WHAT I'VE TOLD YOU

MOVE. GET FIT. HAVE FUN.

YOU CAN ACTUALLY skip the rest of the book and just come here, where I tell you what I told you in the first nine chapters.

Maybe instead of a philosophical conclusion, I should end up with a quiz, like all my old teachers used to do. That way I don't have to figure out how to say anything succinct, witty, and inspiring. How about something like:

1. Did you read the book?
   a. Yes, cover to cover, and I wanted more.
   b. I started it, but then I was so inspired that I had to go out to the gym and work out.
   c. Well . . .
   d. I'm not even reading this book now.

2. Did it make you want to do a triathlon?
   a. I've already signed up, dude!
   b. Wouldn't it be more fun to stand in my garage and hit myself on the head with a hammer?
   c. Well . . .
   d. Maybe when I retire.

3. Did it make you want to rise up and smack me upside my impertinent head?
   a. Yeah, you are kind of a smartass.
   b. I laughed till I peed my Lycra running shorts
   c. No, 'cause I didn't read it.

4. Will you buy copies of this book for all your friends, family, and co-workers?
   a. Can I buy them by the case? [The slow fat triathlete says *yes!*]
   b. If I gave this book to my friends, I wouldn't have any friends left.
   c. Maybe a couple.
   d. Is it OK to give your sister-in-law a book called *Slow Fat Triathlete*?

5. If not, why not?
   a. I'm afraid of my sister-in-law thinking I think she's fat.
   b. I'm afraid my little brother will do a triathlon before I do.

6. You don't want to do a triathlon after reading this book. This is because . . .
   a. I made it sound like hell on earth?
   b. I made it sound like fun, but too difficult?
   c. You don't want to deal with all the equipment?
   d. You don't want to deal with all the training?
   e. You never intended to do one in the first place. You just liked the title?

7. If you are going to do a triathlon, when will you do it?
   a. In the next three months.
   b. In the next six months.
   c. In the next year.
   d. Sometime before I qualify for the senior discount.

8. Which one of these statements do you most agree with?
   a. She's right, you know—you shouldn't worry if you're old or slow or fat or all of the above. You should just go out and do what you want to do.
   b. Slow, fat, and old people are disgusting and should never be let out in public wearing any kind of tight-fitting clothing.
   c. It's better to be slow and fat than to be fat and not moving at all.

OK, enough of this frivolity. Do the quiz and send in your answers to www.slowfattriathlete.com (don't forget the two Ts), I'll grade it and return it with comments. Seriously.

I guess I'm going to have to say something inspiring after all. If you decide not to do a triathlon after reading this book, that's cool. But what I really hope is that the book spurs you to do something with your body and mind that makes an impact on your life. I happen to think that the combination of physical effort, mental discipline, goofy humor, and occasional spiritual wow that triathlon offers me is a great thing that has a supremely positive impact on my life. I'm in the best shape of my life, and I've learned an incredible amount about myself, about my body and my spirit and my will, and about how to put on a wetsuit without falling over. But you might decide to take up outrigger canoeing or tae kwon do or the tango. Or you might decide to take a walk around the block every day. Whatever you do, believe in the beauty of movement, of the intricate and powerful construction of your body, and the unfathomable complexity that links it to your mind and your emotions. You have just as much right to that beauty as everyone else in the world. Reach out and take it.

I hope you do a triathlon, and, having done one, come back again and again and become a full-fledged addict. I hope you get fit and surprise yourself with what you can do. I hope you challenge yourself and learn the truths about yourself that you only learn when you feel like you might not have another step left in you. I hope you meet some incredible people who have great things to teach you and things to learn from you. And most of all, of course, I hope you have fun. Whatever you do. Have fun.

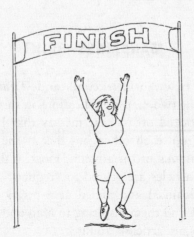

Resources:
A HIGHLY UNSYSTEMATIC LIST OF STUFF THAT MIGHT BE HELPFUL

ORGANIZATIONS

USA Triathlon (www.usatriathlon.org): The governing body of triathlon in the USA. Most races are USAT sanctioned, which means that there's insurance, and the race directors meet the USAT's safety requirements, and there are race officials to make sure that everyone's following the rules and being safe. You can use their Web site to find out triathlon rules, join the organization (saves you nine dollars every time you enter a USAT race), or find a triathlon club.

Team Clydesdale (www.teamclydesdale.com/index2.html) is the "world governing body for Weight Class Athletics," so you can be internationally ranked as a Clydesdale (guys over 200 pounds) or Athena (women over 145 pounds) if you join Team Clydesdale. I haven't joined yet, but that's just because I'm cheap.

MAGAZINES—PRINT

Inside Triathlon (www.insidetri.com) and *Triathlete* (www.triathletemag.com) are the two major publications in this field. I'm sure their editors would be ticked off to hear me say that I find them virtually indistinguishable from each other, but that is the honest truth. They have articles on famous pro triathletes, races, training, nutrition, and gear. Some of the articles are geared to "regular" people, but a lot of them are pretty technical and aimed at a pretty advanced audience. Having said that, I find them inspiring to read and I love looking at all the gear in the ads and articles. Yummy.

ONLINE MAGAZINES AND TRIATHLON WEB SITES

Tri-Newbies Online (www.trinewbies.com): This site has a wealth of information on the usual topics—training, nutrition, gear, etc. One of the best resources here is a series of training plans, from a ten-week plan for a beginner training for a sprint triathlon, to a thirty-six-week Ironman odyssey. They also have very active discussion forums and a great classifieds section. I bought a used bike here at a great price. Of course I still have to get it fitted to my body, but all in good time.

Slowtwitch (www.slowtwitch.com): One of the great patriarchs of the sport, Dan Empfield, is the publisher and guru of this idiosyncratic online mag. Empfield was the founder of Quintana Roo, an equipment company that pioneered triathlon-specific wetsuits and bikes. He's also an experienced race director, age-group racer, and all-around Person to Know in triathlon. Just going back to the Web site to refresh my memory of it, I got caught in two fascinating articles and wasted a solid half hour. Though I find the site's navigation awkward and the content unstructured, I never stop by that URL without learning something good and having a laugh at the same time.

Triathlon Informer (www.triathloninformer.com): A relative newcomer to the online tri medium, Triathlon Informer offers race coverage, features on some of the lesser-known figures in triathlon, a fun "Roadtrip" section, and good, in-depth triathlon writing. Founder and former Slowtwitch editor Amy White loves the sport and knows how to write. To get the full bounty of the Informer, you must subscribe to the e-mail newsletter that arrives in your inbox three times a week. Costs thirty-five dollars per year, but great if you're a tri junkie and just can't get enough triathlon news.

TransitionTimes.com (www.transitiontimes.com) has a few articles, some classifieds, and bulletin boards. Offers a free weekly e-mail newsletter, which I haven't checked out.

HOW TO FIND TRIATHLONS

The American Triathlon Calendar at www.trifind.com. This is a very handy site, especially if you are trying to find races all over the country.

When you get into searching by state the calendar starts to call itself the Triathalator, which I guess it can do if it wants to.

At **Active.com** (www.active.com) you can find races of almost any description from 5K walks to adventure racing, and if the race has linked its registration to Active.com, you can sign up right there online. You can commit yourself to strenuous athletic endeavors without stirring from your desk!

Inside Triathlon. You can check out the race calendar in the print version or go to www.insidetri.com and check out the Web site calendar. The Web site is much more extensive.

Events Online (www.eventsonline.ca) is a useful site for locating triathlons and other athletic events in Canada. (Who says we never think about you guys up there?)

BOOKS

IT'S JUST POSSIBLE that after reading this book, you may want to read more about triathlon. In fact, I would strongly recommend that you do. There are a lot of people out there who have written in much more detail about the sport and have a lot of actual knowledge to share. These are the books that I read before doing my first race:

Triathlon 101: Essentials for Multisport Success, by John Mora (Human Kinetics, 1999). Russ loaned me this book while I was training for my first tri and I still haven't given it back. It's easy to follow, it's sensible, and it's very accessible for beginners. I still refer to John's race-day checklist to make sure I'm not forgetting anything. This is an essential book in any first-timer's library.

Swimming Made Easy, by Terry Laughlin (Swimware, Inc., 2001). A useful piece of writing with photographs and detailed drill descriptions. I think it helped make me a smoother, more relaxed swimmer. I'm still not fast, but becoming smoother and more relaxed is more than half the battle.

I now have a larger collection of triathlon books, and I think you might also want to check these out:

Triathlons for Women, by Sally Edwards (Velo Press, 2002). Now in its third edition, this is a great instructional and informational book for women triathletes. Sally Edwards is a pioneering triathlete and the spokeswoman for the Danskin women's triathlon series. She has good things to say about technique, women's wellness issues, and getting inspired to train. I think she gets into technical matters like heart rate zones a little early for readers who are just looking to start their first triathlon, but this is a great resource nonetheless.

Triathlete's Training Bible, by Joe Friel (Velo Press, 1998). This book is more for intermediate to advanced triathletes who are ready to take their training and performance to the next level. I picked this up as a novice and was completely intimidated by its level of detail and scientific analysis. Having said that, these are the principles my coach uses to train her athletes, and I think they totally work. Joe Friel is a major guru in the triathlon world, so if you like to get geeky, this is the book for you.

Triathlete's Training Diary for Dummies, by Allen St. John (For Dummies, 2001). This book's conversational, light tone makes it easy to digest. It's basically a diary or logbook with some helpful hints for training and racing in the first half. It's a good tool for recording your workouts if you like the old fashioned method of writing things on paper.

Triathloning For Ordinary Mortals, by Steven Jonas (W.W. Norton & Co., 1999). Another really helpful book for folks who are just getting started. Also the only tri book I know that pictures normal-sized athletes on the cover.

PLACES TO BUY STUFF

Tri-Zone (www.tri-zone.com): Lots and lots of triathlon stuff, organized clearly and informally, the way I like it. They have swim stuff, bike stuff, run stuff, and other stuff. What more do you need? Oh, triathlon clothing, of course. They have lots of that, too.

TriSports.com (www.trisports.com): They call themselves a triathlon superstore, and they do have a lot of things. Cleaner layout than Tri-Zone, but much the same sort of thing.

Sports Basement (www.sportsbasement.com): Stuff for cheap. Can't go wrong.

Sierra Trading Post (www.sierratradingpost.com): A huge barn of a site, with a little of almost everything from flannel sheets to bike jerseys. And it's the bike jerseys that interest me. Oh, and the bargains in technical fabric workout gear. Some fantastic deals, especially if you're an odd size or don't mind persimmon-colored running tights.

Junonia (www.junonia.com): This is a very useful site for the slow fat female who wants to get workout clothes, sports bras, and swimsuits that actually fit. Large sizes only, so skinny chicks, don't bother.

Title 9 Sports (www.title9sports.com): Cool athletic clothes for women. The print catalog has a bunch of quotes and profiles from buff but real women who do lots of fun outdoors things. Kinda makes you want to do likewise. Not so good on the large sizes but if you fit into that standard S-XL range, some nice gear here.

Terry Precision Cycling (www.terrybicycles.com): Terry first became known for making quality bicycles specifically designed for a woman's proportions. If you're having trouble getting a bike that fits you, try finding a dealer that stocks Terry. They also sell cool cycling clothes, many available in plus sizes.

Performance Bicycle (www.performancebike.com): An indispensable catalog and Web site for me. They always have stuff you need on sale, and their house brand clothing is good, solid, everyday training wear. You can buy fancy brand-name stuff here, too, if you want to spend money. A good source for sports drinks, gels, bars, etc.

Bike Nashbar (www.nashbar.com): A very similar kind of deal to Performance Bicycle. Everything the gearhead could possibly want, and a lot of stuff that the novice cyclist won't even know what it's for. I use Performance more, but that's because they have a bricks and mortar store not too far from me, which is handy for returns and all.

TherapyZone (www.therapyzone.com): A good place to buy therapeutic equipment like foam rollers, exercise balls, and sticky mats for your stretching and yoga. Remember stretching?

COOL INFORMATION

Total Immersion Swimming: (www.totalimmersion.net) Terry Laughlin's near-mystical system for improving your swimming by making you more "fishlike" in the water. You can get books, tapes, and DVDs here and also sign up for clinics in your area.

Runner's World: (www.runnersworld.com) Runner's World is the total online resource for runners. And even for slow fat triathletes who run. Running FAQs, training plans, shoe information, all kinds of great stuff.

MEDICAL ISSUES

Sports Injury: About.com has a pretty cool section on sports injuries—how to prevent them, or, if you didn't prevent them, how to recognize them and treat them. (http://sportsmedicine.about.com/cs/injuryprevention/)

Athletes with Diabetes: www.diabetesandsports.com has a forum, FAQs, and other resources, hosted by a guy with Type I diabetes who completed Ironman Wisconsin not too long ago. He also hooks up people with and without diabetes to endurance events in their region.

High Blood Pressure: There's a great article at Aetna InteliHealth (http://www.intelihealth.com/IH/ihtIH/WSIHW000/8315/24000/349496.html?d=dmtContent) about how your body responds to exercise and why it's so important for people with high blood pressure. May not be anything you haven't heard before, but to me it seemed like solid information presented in a way that I could understand.

Arthritis: Exercise helps it, the docs say. Maybe running isn't the best thing for your arthritis, but you could be a swim-bike-walk triathlete, or an around-the-block walker, or a century cyclist (100 mile rider). Check out the information at WebMDHealth (http://my.webmd.com/content/article/78/95590) for an introduction to arthritis and diabetes.

ADVENTURE RACING

Never done it, but I intend to. If you find any of these links useful, fun, or harmful, let me know at www.slowfattriathlete.com.

US Adventure Racing Association: (www.usara.com) This is the governing body of adventure racing in the U.S. They feature a calendar of events on their Web site, and a form where you can request information about adventure racing clubs in your area.

Balance Bar Adventure Racing Series: (www.balance.com) Balance sponsors some of the better-known adventure races in the US. I kind of like their energy bars, too.

Muddy Buddy Series: (www.muddybuddy.com) More obstacle course than true "adventure," but lots of fun according to my triclub friends who've done it.

Acknowledgments

MY HUSBAND TIM, my Mom and Dad, and my brother Jonathan all believed I could and should write a book. For that, and for all their unstinting love and support, I thank them every day. Tim also illustrated this book, which is really cool.

Slow Fat Triathlete is about evolving as you move down life's path, and my extraordinary friends make that path pretty darn fun for me: Michelle, a girl's best friend, always. Russ, the catalyst for this endurance sports stuff. Will and Mike, with whom I can just be. Anne, of the amazing mind. Indigo, a blaze of light. Beth, a constant inspiration. Merrin, the book's fairy godmother. Chris, Nan, Sue, Dana, Timo: I thank you for your friendship and for reading my words with such gusto. And David, you made this book happen, to my immeasurable astonishment and gratitude. Keep visualizing.

The Silicon Valley Triathlon Club creates an exuberant and welcoming environment in which to practice the sport of triathlon. Newbies coach Dan Sauers and the fabulous Gina Kehr inspired and coached me when I was a truly slow, fat, nervous beginner. My coach, Lisa Engles, trains my body and mind with science and humor and unshakable belief in what can be. And all my training buddies from Tuesday track, Wednesday open water swims, Thursday bricks, Saturday rides, Sunday runs—you are what it's all about.

The Wonderful Weight Watchers Women of the Friday morning meeting have brought wisdom, humor, and compassion to the best morning of my week. Also, Sara and all the online buddies on the message boards have been a big part of the weight-loss journey. It is a journey well worth the taking, much like an endurance sport. Each tiny step adds up to something big.

Thanks to John Kaemmerling for taking great pictures.
And, finally, thanks to Matthew Lore for laughing out loud.

Index

About the Author

JAYNE WILLIAMS grew up in the halcyon suburbs of Northern California, began her impractical education in Russian literature at Harvard, and got an MA in Slavic Literature from the University of California at Berkeley. She has organized whitewater rafting expeditions in Siberia and around the world, and enjoyed years of frantic poverty as a freelance writer, interpreter, and editor. She has dabbled in public service and the Internet boom/bust, and lives in Mountain View, California, with her husband Tim and their psycho-cat surrogate child.